RHEUMATOLOGY

New Directions in Therapy

EDWARD E. ROSENBAUM, M.D.
Clinical Professor of Medicine
Formerly Chief, Division of Rheumatology
University of Oregon Health Sciences Center
Portland, Oregon

 Medical Examination Publishing Co., Inc.
an Excerpta Medica company

969 Stewart Avenue　　•　　Garden City, New York 11530

notice

The editor(s) and/or author(s) and the publisher of this book have made every effort to ensure that all therapeutic modalities that are recommended are in accordance with accepted standards at the time of publication.

The drugs specified within this book may not have specific approval by the Food and Drug Administration in regard to the indications and dosages that are recommended by the editor(s) and/or author(s). The manufacturer's package insert is the best source of current prescribing information.

Copyright © 1979 by
MEDICAL EXAMINATION
PUBLISHING CO. , INC.
an Excerpta Medica company

Library of Congress Card Number
79-67448

ISBN   0-87488-683-X

October, 1979

Printed in the United States of America

SIMULTANEOUSLY PUBLISHED IN:

Europe   :   HANS HUBER PUBLISHERS
                                   Bern, Switzerland

South and East Asia   :   TOPPAN COMPANY (S) Pte. Ltd.
                                   Singapore

United Kingdom   :   HENRY KIMPTON PUBLISHERS
                                   London, England

Introduction

This book is the summary of over 40 years of personal experience in treating rheumatic diseases and teaching a generation of students.

As a junior medical student in 1936, I encountered my first patient with rheumatoid arthritis. The patient had been hospitalized to demonstrate the disease. Scientific therapy was limited, and the few physicians who treated the disease were frowned upon as quacks. During my internship, I met a German-trained physician who hospitalized patients with rheumatoid arthritis for complete diagnostic studies before starting injections of gold salts. No self-respecting intern associated with him.

University rheumatologists of the early 1940's preached the doctrine of adequate aspirin but utilized bacterial vaccines, artificial fever, killed intravenous typhoid vaccine, bee venom, and large doses of vitamin D in treatment. It was not until the advent of cortisone in 1949 that the treatment of rheumatic disease became respectable, for at last something definitive and dramatic could be done for these patients.

To this day, the treatment of rheumatic diseases leaves much to be desired. We are dealing with chronic diseases of unknown causes; and, by necessity, therapy is nonspecific and often toxic We still do not know the cause of the most common of these diseases. Although current theories provide some basis for research and some rationale for therapy, as yet, no theory has survived for more than a few years. As one 80-year-old patient commented when I explained that osteoarthritis in her knee was due to the wear and tear of life, "Doctor, both my feet were born at the same time. Why is one knee good and one bad?"

Since we are dealing with chronic disease and imperfect results, the art of medicine is particularly important. I once asked a leading rheumatologist to what he attributed his success. "I used to be a used car salesman," was his reply. He was not implying dishonesty or the sale of shoddy merchandise, but was referring to the need for the physician to sell the treatment to the patient.

In general, this book represents the mainstream of current therapy. However, because we can never predict results or toxicity for the individual patient, there are considerable variations among experts in the management of specific problems, and the non-expert occasionally confounds the expert by using an approach that unexpectedly succeeds for a particular patient.

Shortly after indomethacin was approved for general use, rheumatologists debated its value in the treatment of rheumatoid arthritis. Personally, I had never felt that indomethacin was of much value, but it was during this period that I had a particularly frustrating patient with rheumatoid arthritis. Nothing worked! When I returned from my vacation, a young associate informed me that he had started this particular patient on indomethacin—I was furious! Just then our receptionist announced that the patient was on the telephone. "I'll take the call," I snapped to my young colleague; "I hope he has not perforated an ulcer." I announced myself to the patient on the telephone, and he pleaded, "Please let me talk to the real doctor, the one who started me on Indocin."

There are no absolutes in the treatment of rheumatic diseases. Deviation is permissible, if backed by sound logic and reasoned consideration of the risk of toxicity.

Most of the therapy discussed will be drug therapy; however, physiotherapy and occupational therapy are an integral part of treatment (see Part Three, Chapter 4, Physiotherapy).

It should be borne in mind that the rheumatic diseases, even degenerative arthritis, have natural courses of exacerbations and remissions that compound the problems of therapy. If the patient is in the natural remission phase anything works; if in the exacerbation phase, often nothing succeeds.

Approach this book as a guideline; in the treatment of rheumatic diseases, perhaps more than in other medical specialties, there is room for individual judgment.

Contributors

JAMES TODD ROSENBAUM, M.D.
Fellow of the American Rheumatism Association
Fellow in Immunology
Stanford University School of Medicine
Stanford, California

RICHARD BARRY ROSENBAUM, M.D.
Assistant Clinical Professor of Neurology
University of Oregon Health Sciences Center
Portland, Oregon

ROBERT ALAN ROSENBAUM, M.D.
Assistant Clinical Professor of Neurology
University of Oregon Health Sciences Center
Portland, Oregon

Acknowledgments

I am indebted to:

Drs. Phillip Hench and Charles Slocumb, superb teachers who first showed me the way.

The publisher and their editor, Howard Granat, without whose encouragement I never would have started.

Drs. James, Richard, and Robert Rosenbaum who contributed not only individual chapters but important critical reviews of many of the other chapters.

Lois Rosenbaum who helped so much with the editing and correcting of the English style, and her secretary, Laura de Looze, who typed, retyped, and retyped the manuscript so faithfully.

Betty Jones of the Oregon Chapter of the Arthritis and Rheumatism Foundation who was helpful in pointing out the aid to be gotten from the American Rheumatism Association.

To Steve and Laura

*By the time that they are old enough to under-
stand this it will be archaic, but that is what will
make the world a better place to live in.*

Arthritis: Inflammation of a joint.

Rheumatism: An indefinite term applied to various conditions with pain or other symptoms which are of articular origin or related to other elements of the musculoskeletal system.

Stedman's Medical Dictionary

Sometimes when I tell patients that they have rheumatism, they reply, "Thank God I don't have arthritis." If I tell them that they have arthritis, some answer, "Thank God I don't have rheumatism."

Contents

Part One: THE DRUGS

CHAPTER 1: GENERAL PRINCIPLES

The bulk of the drugs used in the treatment of rheumatic diseases are nonspecific. The same drugs are used in treatment of gout as in osteoarthritis and in rheumatoid arthritis. The mode today is to speak of them as being "anti-inflammatory," implying that not only are they analgesic, but they also lessen edema and inflammation. Classification of rheumatic diseases has resulted in some drug specificity, but only in a few cases; nonspecificity results in trial-and-error therapy. The physician first tries a relatively safe drug. If it does not work, he goes to another drug in the same classification or one with greater toxicity.

Because many antirheumatic drugs are toxic, we are faced with the problem of treating a nonfatal disease with a drug that in rare instances may cause death. Drug toxicity has resulted in personal prejudices on the part of treating physicians who often discard one drug for another equally toxic drug. For years the accepted treatment of rheumatoid spondylitis was radiation therapy. It was an excellent treatment until it was discovered that radiated patients had an increased incidence of lymphomas. Phenylbutazone was then substituted and subsequently discarded by many when it produced fatalities secondary to agranulocytosis. In its place, the more toxic Cytoxan was prescribed. Now, as Cytoxan is being discarded, Imuran is being extolled, to be soon replaced by penicillamine and maybe even by levamisole. All of these drugs carry with them serious risk of morbidity and mortality.

Another problem is that many of the drugs are not "approved" for the treatment of the rheumatic diseases. This does not mean that the drugs are ineffective. It means that they have not gone through rigid FDA testing. In treating the rheumatic patient, the physician must constantly evaluate the efficacy-to-toxicity ratio. He must discuss with the patient risks and consequences; and, where the drug is "not approved," he must inform the patient of the experimental nature of the therapy.

1

There is constant pressure on the patient by well-meaning friends and the press to seek new and better treatment; this pressure is transferred to the physician. The physician, much like the psychoanalyst, should repeatedly be asking himself: "Am I treating the patient or am I treating myself?"

One unresolved question is: Can some of these drugs help some patients but make the disease worse in others? I compare the treatment of rheumatic diseases today to the treatment of pneumonia if bacteriology were unknown. We would know that the patient had fever and a consolidated lung, but we would not know if the etiology was staph, strep, or viral; so we would empirically treat with a series of antibiotics, starting with penicillin. Even though we would be helping a number of patients, we would be harming the patient with tuberculosis. No one has seriously addressed himself to this problem regarding the drugs used in the treatment of rheumatic diseases, but I suspect from some of the isolated reports of serious toxic effects that some drugs may actually make the disease worse in some patients.

Two drugs, acetominophen (Tylenol) and propoxyphene (Darvon), often used by arthritics, are not discussed in the drug category. They do have the advantage of not causing gastrointestinal upsets, but propoxyphene has caused habituation and habituation is a constant threat in a chronic disease. Neither of these drugs is anti-inflammatory; their effect is only analgesic and therefore they are not usually included in a discussion of drugs used for rheumatic diseases.

DRUG TOXICITY

The toxicity of the drugs used in the treatment of arthritic diseases presents an ongoing problem for the following reasons:

1. The chronicity of the disease demands long-term therapy.

2. There is a high incidence of drug sensitivity in patients with systemic lupus and rheumatoid arthritis.

3. The toxicities of many of the drugs are similar and, in some instances, additive. Thus, a patient may be on aspirin, Indocin, and prednisone, any of which may cause peptic ulceration.

4. Some of the drugs may actually cause side effects such as myopathy (large doses of prednisone, chloroquine) or peripheral neuritis (gold) which may be indistinguishable from the rheumatic disease.

Because of these problems, I suggest the following rules:

1. Constantly review the package inserts. New side effects are reported that may have escaped your notice. Always consider that the drug may make the patient worse instead of better.

2. If a patient is not doing well, consider stopping the drug, but never withdraw steroids abruptly.

3. Consider any unusual manifestation a side effect until proven otherwise.

4. Avoid mixtures, particularly drugs that have similar side effects.

5. See the patient at regular intervals.

6. At regular intervals, review with the patient all the drugs he is taking. STOP the unnecessary ones.

7. If the patient is on chloroquine or hydroxychloroquin (Plaquenil), review with the patient at each visit when the next eye check is due.

8. Do not refill any of the toxic drugs over the telephone.

9. Do not prescribe toxic drugs to an uncooperative patient.

10. Insist on regular laboratory tests as indicated. Do not be deterred from performing necessary tests by insurance carriers, economists, and politicians. They are not the ones sued for malpractice.

11. Avoid drugs in pregnancy and in lactating mothers.

REFERENCE

1. Buckingham, R.B.: Interactions involving antirheumatic agents. Bulletin on Rheumatic Diseases, Part I. 28:960, Part II. 28:966, 1978.

CHAPTER 2: THE MYTH OF ASPIRIN

Rheumatologists traditionally start their lectures with the statement, "Aspirin is the drug of choice in the treatment of rheumatic diseases and the accepted standard against which other anti-inflammatory agents are measured."

Aspirin is no longer a trade name. It is derived from acetyl plus spiraeic acid* and refers to acetylsalicylic acid.[1]

As some skill is required in the proper use of aspirin, its background is worth a brief review. The ancient Greeks recognized that willow bark was medicinal. This seemed logical for, as everyone knows, anything bitter has to be therapeutic. In 1827 the bitter glucoside salicin was extracted from tree bark and ultimately yielded salicylic acid. It was found that salicylic acid could also be prepared from oil of gaultheria (oil of wintergreen) and from phenol. The salt produced was sodium salicylate and was used in 1875 as an antipyretic and to treat rheumatic fever.[2]

Felix Hofman, a German chemist, synthesized acetylsalicylic acid (aspirin) for use by his father, who had rheumatoid arthritis, and Hofman's director, Dresser, introduced the new drug, which he named aspirin, into medical practice.[3,4] Three quarters of a century later, we pay lip service to the benefits of aspirin, but in practice few patients or physicians rely on aspirin, as the sole drug.[5]

The doctor who prescribes aspirin as the sole therapy for a chronic rheumatic condition is doomed to failure. The patient, frightened by the chronicity of the disease, has already been advised by radio, television, and newspaper to take aspirin. To the sufferer, it does not make sense to spend time and money with a doctor only to receive the exact advice previously received free from the media. The doctor may know that aspirin works, but the patient simply does not believe in its efficacy. Unless educated by the physician, the compliance with aspirin therapy of the average chronic disease patient is poor.[6]

* An obsolete name for salicylic acid.

Since its introduction, aspirin has received worldwide acceptance as the safest and most widely used analgesic. What originally began as a simple analgesic agent has become a complicated
therapeutic modality. Because of aspirin's widespread use, over
200 different aspirin preparations plus innumerable mixtures and
similar salts are available in the United States. The choice of
which preparation to use can in itself be a formidable problem. [7]

Aspirin is absorbed rapidly from the stomach and the duodenum.
If a reliable brand is used, blood levels are detectable within a
few minutes and absorption is completed in two to four hours.
The rate of absorption is largely determined by the physical
characteristics of the tablet that is administered. In the body,
aspirin is rapidly hydrolyzed in the serum and conjugated in the
liver by glycine and glucuronide. The conjugation with glycine
has a maximum rate which in the average patient can be achieved
with less than two tablets of aspirin. This explains why one or
two tablets of aspirin can be the difference between therapeutic
success and toxicity. The body can handle only a limited amount
of aspirin at a time. [8]

The conjugates of aspirin are excreted in the urine. Many factors influence the rate of excretion and the rate of absorption,
including the pH of the stomach, the pH of the urine, the physical activity of the patient, the diet, and competing drugs. In the
plasma, salicylates are bound to protein, particularly serum albumin. This may explain the difficulty, noted by many clinicians,
in obtaining therapeutic salicylate levels in some patients with
severe rheumatoid arthritis who have impairments in their protein metabolism. This fact also represents a theoretical contraindication to the combined use of salicylates and many of the so-
called newer anti-inflammatory drugs which are also bound to
the serum albumin. [9]

The peak concentration of salicylates in the plasma after con-
sumption of two aspirin tablets occurs in two hours; the half-life
is in the neighborhood of five hours in the average patient. Almost all ingested salicylates are eliminated in the urine within
48 hours. [10]

In the human subject, if one compares two regular aspirin tablets (650 mg) with one sustained-release aspirin tablet (1300 mg),
one notes that the sustained-release tablet has a sustained salicylate level at eight hours, while the standard aspirin tablet
must be repeated in four hours to achieve this level of salicylate.
However, if one administers four standard tablets (1300 mg) at
the same time as one 1300 mg sustained-release tablet, the

salicylate level in eight hours is the same. The administration of four tablets, as compared to one sustained-release tablet has the advantage of a higher salicylate level in the early hours.[11]

The half-life of a standard aspirin tablet (325 mg) is two and one-half hours which increases to seven hours after administration of four tablets and which approaches 20 hours following a dose of 10 to 20 grams. The maximum therapeutic response from high dose aspirin requires about one week. In other words, when high doses of aspirin are used, a "steady state" is not reached in less than five to seven days.[12,13]

Clinicians have long recognized that the anti-inflammatory effect of aspirin is achieved only when administered in its maximum tolerated level. Traditionally, this level was recognized by a buzzing sensation in the patient's ears. At best, this is a rough guide and a poor substitute for laboratory tests of serum salicylate levels.

Not until 1952 was it demonstrated objectively that aspirin was anti-inflammatory when used in large doses in rheumatic fever.[14]

In 1965, Fremont-Smith and Bayles first objectively demonstrated a fact that clinicians had long suspected - that aspirin is an anti-inflammatory agent whose anti-inflammatory effect is not achieved unless the largest tolerated dose of aspirin is used. In their original tests, these investigators used Bufferin around the clock. The final total aspirin dosage ranged from 3.6 to 7.5 grams in 24 hours. The average dose was 5.2 grams.[15]

The anti-inflammatory effect of aspirin is dose-related. Dosage in the range of two tablets every four hours has no anti-inflammatory action.[16]

It appears, then, that aspirin is a rapidly absorbed and rapidly excreted drug whose short half-life in the body can be increased by using three or four tablets in a single dose and by administering it at four-hour intervals. In this program, a stable level or "steady state" is reached in about one week. Because of the limited enzyme capacity in the liver where aspirin is conjugated, one or two tablets in a 24-hour period can be the difference between success and failure or the difference between a therapeutic dose and a toxic level. To treat a patient successfully with aspirin, I suggest the following program:

1. Convince the patient that aspirin will work. Advise him that the prescribed dose should be taken at four-hour intervals

around the clock without regard to the presence of pain. The aspirin is being taken primarily to relieve stiffness and swelling, thus requiring an unusually large dose.

2. Decide whether to use a good standard brand aspirin tablet, a buffered aspirin tablet (Ascriptin or Bufferin) or coated aspirin (Lilly's enseals, Ecotrin). The advantage of plain aspirin is that it is the least expensive. Buffered aspirin tends to have better patient acceptance; coated aspirin is the best tolerated but introduces the problem of erratic absorption.[7] The physician must be aware of the various problems with these different preparations and must select the preparations that best fit his skills and the patient's needs. Involvement with mixtures is not advantageous and, traditionally, salts such as sodium salicylate are not as effective as plain aspirin. The standard teaching that aspirin is preferred to sodium salicylate is based on historical and theoretical experience.[18,19,20]

3. Every third day the blood salicylate level should be drawn. The aim is to achieve a blood salicylate level of 20-30 mg percent. The dosage is increased by only two tablets in a 24-hour period until the therapeutic level is reached. Once the therapeutic level is reached, the dosage is maintained indefinitely, bearing in mind that extraneous factors, such as ketosis, weight reduction diets, other drugs, fever, and diarrhea may cause alterations in the blood salicylate level.

4. The patient on saturated doses of aspirin must be warned not to take over-the-counter preparations. Currently, there are at least 200 products on the market containing aspirin, most of which are in combination.[21] Aspirin, particularly in the dosage level suggested, is not an innocuous drug. Gastrointestinal disturbances are the most common adverse reactions. These can range from nausea, vomiting, indigestion, occult bleeding and frank peptic ulcer. Hepatitis and thrombocytopenia are rare complications. Tinnitus and hearing loss can be the initial common signs of toxicity, but they are not a reliable index. A small percentage of patients is hypersensitive to aspirin and may develop a rash or a life-threatening asthmatic-type anaphylactic reaction. Urticaria may also occur. Aspirin interferes with the prothrombin determination and with the uricosuric effect of many drugs.[22]

To counteract the problems of gastrointestinal distress and of the need of frequent dosages, two forms of aspirin have been recently reintroduced: salicyl-salicylic acid (Disalcid) and choline magnesium trisalicylate (Trilisate). These older forms of aspirin probably never achieved popularity because their long half-life offered no advantage as simple analgesics. They do offer an advantage over the standard aspirin tablet in that they are much less prone to cause GI distress and do not have to be administered as frequently as aspirin to achieve therapeutic blood levels. The recommended starting dose of Disalcid is two tablets three times a day and the starting dose of Trilisate is one tablet twice a day, increasing or decreasing the dose as needed. One should realize that these drugs, being reintroductions of old salicylates, have not been subjected to critical double-blind studies that some of the newer anti-inflammatory drugs have been. They do, however, seem to have good patient acceptance and should be carefully evaluated as a possible substitute for the standard aspirin.

Aspirin today, when properly used, is the least expensive and best quick-acting anti-inflammatory agent that we have. Its proper administration, however, requires as much skill and patient compliance as does the administration of insulin to a diabetic.

SUMMARY

Aspirin comes as a standard 325 mg tablet. In small doses it is analgesic, but it is anti-inflammatory only in doses over 12 tablets a day. To be maximally effective, a blood level of 20-30 mg percent should be reached.

Disadvantages include GI upsets and buzzing in the ears. The necessity of frequent doses and many tablets is also disadvantageous in lessening patient compliance.

Ascriptin is more acceptable to many patients, although more costly, due to the addition of magnesium carbonate, which decreases GI disturbance. In a few patients, large doses of the magnesium may have a laxative effect.

Ecotrin and ASA Enseals are coated aspirins which seldom cause GI upset. However, all the other aspirin problems remain and erratic absorption can occur.

Salicyl-salicylic acid (Disalcid) and choline magnesium trisalicylate (Trilisate) are old compounds in a new dress. In the past we have discarded them as being not as effective an analgesic as aspirin. Because they are less prone to cause GI distress and have better patient acceptance (requiring fewer tablets to produce a therapeutic salicylate level), they are worth consideration.

REFERENCES

1. Vandan, D.: Analgetic drugs - the mild analgetics. Drug Therapy 1:9 The New England Journal of Medicine 1972-1974.

2. Woodbury, D.M.: The salicylates. In: The Pharmacological Basis of Therapeutics. Macmillan Publishing Co., New York, 1975, p. 326.

3. Dresser, H.: Pharmacologishes uber aspirin (Acetysaure). Pflugers archiv fur die gesamte physiologie des menchen undertiere 76:306, 1899.

4. Champion, G.D., et al.: Salicylates in rheumatoid arthritis. In: Clinics in Rheumatic Disease. W.B. Saunders Co., Philadelphia, 1975.

5. Lee, P., et al.: Observations on drug prescribing in rheumatoid arthritis. British Medical Journal 1:424, 1974.

6. Feerstein, J.R., et al.: Patient noncompliance within the context of seeking medical care for arthritis. Journal of Chronic Diseases 26:689, 1973.

7. Is all aspirin alike? Medical Letter 16:57, 1974.

8. Schachter, D. and Morris, J.G.: Salicylate and salicyl conjugates: Fluorimetric estimation, biosynthesis and renal excretion in man. Journal of Clinical Investigation 37:800, 1958.

9. Fremont-Smith, K.: Proceedings of the conference on chronic salicylate administration. Department of Health, Education, and Welfare, Washington, D.C., 1966, pp. 1-5.

10. Wood, P.H.N.: Salicylates. Bulletin on Rheumatic Diseases 12:297, 1965.

11. Leonards, J.R.: Proceedings of the conference on chronic salicylate administration. Department of Health, Education, and Welfare, Washington, D.C., 1966, pp. 8-9.

12. Levy, G.: Pharmacokinetics of salicylate elimination on man. Journal of Pharmaceutical Sciences 54:959, 1965.

13. Levy, G. and Tsuchiy, A.: Salicylate accumulation kinetics in man. The New England Journal of Medicine 287:430, 1972.

14. Fischel, F.R.: Observations on the treatment of rheumatic fever with salicylates, ACTH, and cortisone. Medicine 31: 331, 1952.

15. Fremont-Smith, K., et al.: Salicylate therapy in rheumatoid arthritis. Journal of the American Medical Association 192:1133, 1965.

16. Boardman, et al.: Clinical measurements of the anti-inflammatory effect of salicylates in rheumatoid arthritis. British Medical Journal 4:264, 1967.

17. Collier, H.O.J.: A pharmacological analysis of aspirin. Advances in Pharmacology and Chemotherapy 7:333, 1969.

18. Ferreira, S.H. and Vane, J.R.: New aspects of the mode of action of nonsteroidal anti-inflammatory drugs. Annual Review of Pharmacology 14:57, 1974.

19. Champion, G.P., et al.: Salicylates in rheumatoid arthritis. In: Clinics in Rheumatic Diseases. W.B. Saunders Co., Philadelphia, 1975, p. 250.

20. Leist, E.R. and Banwell, J.G.: Products containing aspirin. The New England Journal of Medicine 291:710, 1974.

21. AMA Drug Evaluation, 3rd ed., AMA Dept. of Drugs, P.S.G. Publishing Co., Littleton, 1977, p. 380.

CHAPTER 3:   PHENYLBUTAZONE AND OXYPHENBUTAZONE

When phenylbutazone (Azolid, Butazolidin) was introduced into the United States in 1952, it was hailed as a new wonder drug.[1] However, when reports of agranulocytosis were published,[2] the drug became unpopular and many physicians still will not prescribe it.[3]

Subsequently, a metabolyte, oxyphenbutazone (Oxalid, Tandearil), was introduced, but there has never been substantial evidence of any advantage in its use.

The drug is a derivative of phenacetin and is closely related to amidopyrine and antipyrine; it is probable that its serious toxic effects are dose-related. When originally introduced, the dosage was up to 1200 mg daily; currently, the accepted dosage ranges from 100 to 400 mg daily.[4]

Phenylbutazone is a potent anti-inflammatory agent and is described as being effective in acute flairs of rheumatoid arthritis, spondylitis, osteoarthritis, and gout.

The package insert lists a number of serious toxic reactions and specifically states that it should not be used for longer than seven days by patients over 60 years of age.

In my experience, phenylbutazone is the most effective drug currently available for the treatment of spondylitis, osteoarthritis, and gout. Because of its toxicity, I do not recommend it as a first line of treatment, but when the other drugs have failed and where the symptoms merit it, it can be a valuable tool.

In my experience, the toxicity has been no worse than most of the other drugs used in the treatment of rheumatic diseases. I recommend the following rules:

1. Decide whether to use phenylbutazone or oxyphenbutazone. There is no point in using both.

11

2. Advise the patient of potential toxicity and tell the patient to discontinue the drug at once if any of the following symptoms develop:
   a) Fever
   b) Sore mouth
   c) Itch
   d) Rash
   e) Heartburn, indigestion, diarrhea, nausea
   f) Edema

3. Do not exceed a dose of 100 mg four times a day after meals and at bedtime with food or milk.

4. If the patient does not obtain unquestionable relief in one week, discontinue use.

5. Do not mix the drug. Do not use it with gold, antimalarials, anticoagulants, or steroids.

6. Keep the maintenance dose at the lowest possible effective dose, 100 to 300 mg daily.

7. Do a complete blood count and urine analysis in one week and every four weeks thereafter.

8. Do not use in patients with congestive heart failure or edema.

The major side effects are:

1. Peptic ulcer: perforation and hemorrhage
2. Bone marrow depression
3. Rash
4. Fluid retention
5. Gastrointestinal upset, particularly peptic ulcer
6. Allergic reactions
7. Thyroid inhibition
8. Renal damage
9. Possible side effects on eyes and ears

In my opinion, phenylbutazone is the most effective of all the anti-inflammatory drugs, with the possible exception of indomethacin. It is ironic that rheumatologists condemn phenylbutazone for its toxicity, then use drugs of equal toxicity such as gold, Cytoxan, azathioprine and penicillamine. Marrow toxicity occurs with an estimated frequency of 1:66,000 prescriptions.[5] This compares favorably with the toxicity of penicillin, total hip replacement, azathioprine, cyclophosphamide, and gold.

SUMMARY

Phenylbutazone and oxyphenylbutazone are chemically related. They are excellent drugs in osteoarthritis, rheumatoid spondylitis, gout, and some patients with rheumatoid arthritis or systemic lupus. They come as a 100 mg tablet and the usual dose is 100 mg to 400 mg daily. The minimum maintenance dose should be established as quickly as possible. The major side effect is the development of peptic ulcer. The severe reported side effect of agranulocytosis has made it unpopular with some physicians. If properly monitored and if the patient is properly instructed, the risk should not be unreasonable.

REFERENCES

1. Kuzell, W.C., et al.: Phenylbutazone (Butazolidin) in rheumatoid arthritis and gout. Journal of the American Medical Association 149:729, 1952.

2. Mauer, E.F.: The toxic effects of phenylbutazone (Butazolidin). The New England Journal of Medicine 253:404, 1955.

3. Hollingsworth, J.W.: Management of Rheumatoid Arthritis and its Complications. Year Book Medical Publishers, Chicago, 1978, p. 52.

4. Kantor, T.G.: Anti-inflammatory drugs. In: Rheumatic Diseases, Katz, W. (ed.), J.B. Lippincott Co., Philadelphia, 1977, p. 881.

5. Girwood, R.H.: Death after taking medicaments. British Medical Journal 1:501, 1974.

CHAPTER 4:   INDOMETHACIN

Indomethacin (Indocin) was introduced in the United States in 1965. It is an indole acetic acid compound with anti-inflammatory activity.[1] Its efficacy in rheumatoid arthritis is debatable but generally accepted.[2] It is very effective in treating spondylitis, gout, and osteoarthritis.

The major problem with indomethacin is the closeness between therapeutic and toxic dosage. Gastrointestinal irritation with peptic ulceration is one of its major side effects. Psychotropic effects, dizziness, headaches, edema, and weight gain are also troublesome side effects.

The usual dose is 25 mg two or three times a day, taken after meals. This may be increased up to 50 mg four times a day if necessary. The higher the dose, the greater the toxicity.

A dosage of 50 to 100 mg at bedtime has been recommended as a preventative for morning stiffness.[3]

The incidence of side effects with long-term indomethacin use is similar to the incidence in patients receiving phenylbutazone, but the side effects are much less likely to be fatal.[4]

The most common side effects, gastrointestinal disturbance, nausea, peptic ulcer, and central nervous system effects, are all serious hazards. Headaches, lightheadedness, dizziness, and confusion are often serious enough to necessitate stopping the drug. Hypersensitivity reactions, retinal changes, and corneal deposits have also been reported.

Indomethacin is an excellent drug when properly used and monitored. Its only limitation is its toxicity.

SUMMARY

Indomethacin comes as a 25 mg and 50 mg capsule. The usual dose ranges from 25 mg to a maximum of 200 mg a day. The minimum maintenance dose, however, should be found as soon as possible. It is an excellent drug in the treatment of osteoar-thritis, rheumatoid spondylitis, and in some cases of rheumatoid arthritis and systemic lupus. Its major limiting side effect is the development of peptic ulcers. It may also cause headache and central nervous system symptoms in susceptible patients.

REFERENCES

1. Famacy, J.P., et al.: Biological effects of nonsteroidal anti-inflammatory drugs. Seminar Arthritis and Rheuma-tism 5:63, 1975.

2. O'Brien, W.M.: Indomethacin: A survey of clinical trials. Clinical Pharmacy and Therapy 9:94, 1968.

3. Huskisson, E.C., et. al.: Evening indomethacin in the treat-ment of rheumatoid arthritis. Annals of Rheumatic Disease 29:393, 1970.

4. Girdwood, R.H.: Death after taking medicaments. British Medical Journal 1:501, 1974.

CHAPTER 5: THE NEWER ANTI-INFLAMMATORY DRUGS

"Newer is not necessarily better."

In recent years a new series of drugs has been introduced into the practice of rheumatology and presented as being as effective as, but safer than, aspirin. At the present time five of these drugs are currently available for clinical use in the United States; it is estimated that 200 similar type drugs are being studied or used throughout the world.[2] The drugs currently approved for clinical use in this country are ibuprofin (Motrin), fenoprofen calcium (Nalfon), naproxen (Naprosyn), tolmetin sodium (Tolectin), and sulindac (Clinoril).

Three of these drugs, ibuprofin (Motrin), fenoprofen calcium (Nalfon), and naproxen (Naprosyn) are similar chemically, being derivatives of proprionic acid. The fourth drug, tolmetin sodium (Tolectin), is a pyrrole compound chemically related to indomethacin, but its pharmacological action is similar to the first three drugs. The fifth drug, sulindac (Clinoril), is the newest drug to be introduced and is an indene derivative and chemically related to indomethacin. It seems to differ, however, in its pharmacological properties from indomethacin in that while it is effective as an antipyretic and anti-inflammatory agent, it does not have the gastrointestinal and central nervous system side effects that indomethacin has.[2,3]

Ibuprofen (Motrin) was the first of the drugs to be introduced into this country and because of this has enjoyed wide popularity. It comes as a 300, 400 and 600 mg tablet. The usual dose is 400 mg, starting with one tablet three times a day and increasing the dose as necessary up to 2400 mg daily.

Naproxen (Naprosyn) has a longer half-life than ibuprofen (Motrin) so that it can be administered every 12 hours. It is available as a 250 mg tablet and is usually prescribed one tablet twice a day. However, as many as three tablets a day may be administered; in such cases it is customary to give one tablet in the morning and two in the evening.

Fenoprofen (Nalfon) has a short half-life. It is available as a 300 or 600 mg tablet and the dosage ranges between 1600 and 2400 mg given in three or four divided doses.

Sulindac (Clinoril) comes as a 150 mg and 200 mg tablet. The usual dosage is 300 to 400 mg daily, usually given as one tablet twice a day.

Since these drugs are closely bound to serum proteins, there is little rationale in exceeding the manufacturer's recommended dose, as larger doses do not seem to increase their effectiveness. Theoretically, since aspirin is also bound to serum protein, it does not appear logical to mix these drugs with aspirin. Some clinicians, however, believe that using these drugs combined with aspirin may have a synergistic effect. Although three of the drugs are very similar chemically, there have been repeated suggestions that if one does not work, it is worth trying the others.[1]

These drugs have been embraced by practicing physicians because they seem to produce fewer side effects and are widely accepted and well tolerated by the patient. However, they have not eliminated all side effects. Gastrointestinal complaints are common, peptic ulcers do occur, and fluid retentions and rashes have been reported. Toxicity is a question of time and dosage. It is premature to be certain of the absolute safety of these drugs. Some serious side effects such as thrombocytopenia with fenoprofen (Nalfon),[4] meningitis with ibuprofen (Motrin),[5] and anaphylactic reactions with Tolectin[6] have been reported. Side effects of tolmetin (Tolectin) are largely gastrointestinal and occur in 30 percent of the patients, but they do not necessarily demand discontinuing treatment. Other side effects include rashes, edema, headaches, and dizziness.[7] Sulindac (Clinoril) seems to have very few side effects. Actually, fewer side effects have been reported with sulindac than with aspirin. Sulindac occasionally causes nausea and dermatitis. Peptic ulcer is rare. To the best of my knowledge, thus far, sulindac has shown no clinically significant interaction with oral anticoagulants or oral hypoglycemic agents, nor has there been any reported case of agranulocytosis following the use of sulindac. Sulindac has been approved for the treatment of osteoarthritis, rheumatoid arthritis, ankylosing spondylitis, the acute painful shoulder, and acute gouty arthritis, but it is a mild inhibitor of platelet function so patients on anticoagulants should be carefully monitored.

As far as is known, these drugs do not alter the course of the disease. Their main value is their anti-inflammatory and analgesic effects. All of these drugs have been reported to be as effective as aspirin in the treatment of rheumatoid arthritis. However, for the most part they have been compared to a fixed, not a variable, dose of aspirin, and this is as valid as comparing a new hypoglycemic agent to a fixed dose of insulin. Increasing the dose of aspirin to its maximum safe dose improves its anti-inflammatory effect. Increasing the dose of the proprionic acid derivatives above the recommended dosage offers no lasting benefit.[7,8]

The major value of these new agents is that they are better accepted by the patient and more easily administered by the physician than aspirin. Many patients do not tolerate aspirin and those that do object to the gastrointestinal symptoms and tinnitus that accompanies large doses of aspirin. It is difficult to obtain patient compliance in taking a large number of pills in a 24-hour period. The primary disadvantage of these drugs is their relatively mild anti-inflammatory action and their cost.

To the practicing physician, these drugs are particularly valuable because they offer a way to conservatively treat a rheumatic disease, avoiding harm to the patient, and obtaining patient compliance.

There is no drug of choice among these five drugs. The initial choice as to which to use depends on each individual's personal experience and preference. My recommendation is to start with sulindac (Clinoril) 200 mg twice a day. This offers the advantage of easy patient compliance, minimum side effects, and the greatest number of approved indications. I would try the Clinoril for a minimum of two weeks and preferably four weeks. If it is not effective, then I would use naproxen (Naprosyn) because it too offers the advantage of twice a day dosage. After a trial of naproxen (Naprosyn), then my order of preference would be ibuprofen (Motrin), fenoprofen (Nalfon), and tolmetin (Tolectin).

This order of sequence simply represents my own personal prejudices, and any physician has a valid right to use these in any sequence that has proved best in his experience.

SUMMARY

The most recently introduced approved anti-inflammatory drugs are ibuprofen (Motrin), fenoprofen calcium (Nalfon), naproxen (Naprosyn), tolmetin sodium (Tolectin), and sulindac (Clinoril). The first three of these drugs are similar chemically: the fourth and fifth drugs are closer chemically to indomethacin. These drugs do have anti-inflammatory and analgesic effects. Some patients will respond to one and not the other. Therefore, it is worthwhile trying all of these drugs in the same patient. Because of their chemical similarity, there is little point in mixing ibuorpfen (Motrin), fenoprofen (Nalfon), and naproxen (Naprosyn). Some clinicians believe that the addition of tolmetin (Tolectin) or Clinoril to the first three may be synergistic. This is not an approved combination and one enters the field of unknown toxicity. Theoretically, aspirin should not be combined with these drugs, but many clinicians do use aspirin feeling that the combination is synergistic.

REFERENCES

1. Meeting of the American Society for Clinical Pharmacology and Therapeutics, Atlanta, Ga., March 1978.

2. Scheebel, A.L.: Nonsteroidal anti-inflammatory drugs. Post graduate Medicine 63:69, 1978.

3. Clinoril (Sulindac) in the management of many arthritic disorders. Merck, Sharp & Dohme, West Point, Pa., 1978.

4. Simpson, R.E., et al.: Acute thrombocytopenia associated with fenoprofen (Letter). The New England Journal of Medicine 298:629, 1978.

5. Widener, H.L., et al.: Ibuprofen-induced meningitis in systemic lupus erythematosus. Journal of the American Medical Association 239:1062, 1978.

6. Restiud, C., et al.: Anaphylaxis from tolmetin. Journal of the American Medical Association 240:246, 1978.

7. Huskinsson, E.C.: Anti-inflammatory drugs. Seminars in Arthritis 7:1, 1977.

8. Wilkens, R.F., et al.: Combination therapy with naproxen and aspirin in rheumatoid arthritis. Arthritis and Rheumatism 19:667, 1976.

CHAPTER 6: CHLOROQUINE AND HYDROXYCHLOROQUINE

"Being crippled is bad enough, but a blind cripple?"

an Ophthalmologist

During World War II, quinine, a military necessity for the troops in the tropics, was scarce. The Germans succeeded in synthesizing the antimalarial chloroquine. The secret of the synthesizing process became known to the Allies, who used chloroquine and its derivatives as a prophylaxis against malaria. It was administered to thousands of people with no known serious consequences, but the dosage used for malarial prophylaxis never approached the dosage used in the treatment of rheumatic diseases.[1]

I first became acquainted with chloroquine in 1950 when I noted that patients of a colleague (Dr. Robert Rinehart) were faring better than mine. On the theory that rheumatoid arthritis was due to amebiases, he had started many of his patients on a course of amebacides, one of which was chloroquine.

By 1954 reports had appeared in literature of the excellent results with chloroquine in rheumatoid arthritis and later in systemic lupus.[2,3,4] Physicians began to use chloroquine in the treatment of rheumatic diseases in doses ten times higher than had been used in the prophylaxis of malaria.

In 1957 a case of chloroquine retinopathy was described,[5] but the report was ignored. By 1958 it was recognized that chloroquine deposits occurred in the cornea. The condition is reversible and has never been considered a serious complication.[6] By 1960 a sufficient number of reports of irreversible retinal damage and blindness had appeared to alert the profession. The resulting malpractice suits, most of which were won by the plaintiffs, practically eliminated the use of chloroquine as a form of therapy,[7,8,9] and subsequent reports of blindness occurring years after discontinuation of the drug almost doomed it to oblivion.[10]

20

The persistence of a few brave souls who demonstrated that to a large extent any toxicity was the result of excessive doses over prolonged periods of time and that the risk of usage in controlled doses was not unreasonable saved the drug.[11,12,13] The importance of warning the patient to discontinue the drug if visual disturbances developed and to have regular ophthalmologic checks for changes in visual fields, scotomata, and loss of color vision (especially red)[11,12] at three- to six-month intervals was recognized. Today, many rheumatologists still refuse to use the drug under any circumstances.[14]

The few double-blind studies of chloroquine's efficacy that have been conducted demonstrate its effectiveness.[15,16,17]

The following discussion represents 28 years of personal experience in the use of chloroquine.

Chloroquine in the United States exists in two forms, chloroquine phosphate, originally marketed as Aralen, and hydroxychloroquine sulfate (Plaquenil). Chloroquine phosphate comes as a 250 mg tablet and hydroxychloroquine as a 200 mg tablet. Chloroquine phosphate 250 mg and hydroxychloroquine sulfate 400 mg (2 tablets) are considered equivalent doses, both producing 150 mg of chloroquine base.[17] As Aralen has not been marketed since 1970, chloroquine phosphate may not be available in some pharmacies. Most rheumatologists prefer the hydroxychloroquine to chloroquine because the former is generally considered less toxic but equally effective. This has not been my personal experience; I have found chloroquine to be more effective, but also probably more toxic.

Emphasis has been placed on blindness that may follow the use of chloroquine, but there are other less serious side effects limiting its use, including gastrointestinal disturbances, nausea, anorexia, and weight loss. These effects can be sufficiently severe to necessitate discontinuation of the drug. Other side effects include dermatitis, convulsions, peripheral neuritis, pigmentation of the skin, and change in hair color, particularly in redheads.[19]

Chloroquine can be used with reasonable safety if the following rules are followed:

1. The diagnosis of rheumatoid arthritis or systemic lupus should be firmly established.

2. Conservative, less toxic drugs should have failed.

3. The patient should be informed and advised to discontinue the drug if visual disturbances such as photophobia, halos around lights, or diplopia appear.

4. An ophthalmologist should check the patient before starting therapy and at three- to six-month intervals as long as the patient is on therapy.

5. The adult dosage should never exceed 250 mg of chloroquine once per day, or 200 mg of hydroxychloroquine (Plaquenil) twice a day.

THE DOSAGE SCHEDULE

Before starting therapy, advise the patient that chloroquine is not an analgesic and that results should not be expected in less than 30 to 90 days. If satisfactory results do not occur in 90 days, there is little point in continuing the drug. Start with chloroquine sulfate, 250 mg once a day after the evening meal. If good results are obtained within 90 days, continue on the once-a-day dosage schedule to six tablets per week, skipping Sunday. If control is maintained, stay on the reduced schedule. If control is not maintained, go back to 250 mg per day. Every six months, attempt to reduce the dose 250 mg per week. Unless toxicity is present, never stop the drug completely. Complete cessation results in eventual exacerbation and the drug is seldom as effective the second time around. The principle is to reduce the dose every six months (one tablet per week) to find the minimum effective dose and never to exceed one tablet per day. If a question of eye toxicity arises, stop the chloroquine. If the chloroquine is not tolerated because of minor toxic effects, Plaquenil, 200 mg twice a day, may be substituted. Plaquenil, however, should not be substituted for chloroquine in case of eye toxicity. The principle of adjusting dosage of Plaquenil is the same as that of chloroquine. Every six months, attempt to lower the dose of Plaquenil. Never exceed a daily dose of 400 mg a day.

In my experience, if either chloroquine or Plaquenil is effective but does not completely control the disease, gold therapy can be added and will often have a synergistic effect.

Recent reports indicate the ophthalmologic safety of long-term hydroxychloroquine treatment and/or chloroquine if proper precautions are taken.[20,21]

SUMMARY

CHLOROQUINE

Chloroquine is available as chloroquine phosphate 250 mg tablets or hydroxychloroquine sulfate (Plaquenil) 200 mg tablets.

SIDE EFFECTS

The major side effect is blindness due to chloroquine combining with retinal pigment. Other side effects are gastrointestinal upset, skin pigmentation, weight loss, peripheral neuritis, and convulsions.

Hydroxychloroquine (Plaquenil) is the one usually used; it is probably less toxic but not as effective as chloroquine phosphate.

DOSAGE

1.   Chloroquine phosphate 250 mg daily
2.   Hydroxychloroquine 200 mg b.i.d.
3.   It may take up to 90 days for a result.
4.   Attempt dose reduction every six months.

PRECAUTIONS

1.   Do not exceed recommended dose.
2.   Inform patient of toxicity.
3.   Have ophthalmologist follow patient.
4.   Do not refill over the phone.
5.   STOP whenever there are any visual complaints or question of eye toxicity.
6.   The above dosage schedule does not apply to children.

REFERENCES

1.   Nylander, U.: Ocular damage in chloroquine therapy. Acta Ophthalmologica (Copenhagen):Supplement 92:5, 1967.

2.   Pillsbury, D.M. and Jacobson, C.: Treatment of chronic discoid lupus erythematosus with chloroquine (Aralen). Journal of the American Medical Association 154:1330, 1954.

3.   Page, E.: Treatment of rheumatoid arthritis with mepacrine. Lancet 2:755, 1954.

4. Diaz-Jouanen, E., et al.: Systemic lupus erythematosus presenting as paniculitis (lupus profundus). Annals of Internal Medicine 82:376, 1975.

5. Cambiaggi, A.: Unusual ocular lesions in a case of systemic lupus erythematosus. A.M.A. Archives of Ophthalmology 57:451, 1957.

6. Calkins, L.L.: Corneal epitheliar changes occurring during chloroquine therapy. Archives of Ophthalmology 60: 981, 1958.

7. Goldman, L., et al.: Reactions to chloroquine observed during treatment of various dermatological disorders. American Journal of Tropical Medicine 6:654, 1959.

8. Hobbs, H.E., et al.: A retinopathy following chloroquine therapy. Lancet 2:478, 1959.

9. Wells, A.G.: Amblyopia in lupus erythematosus. Procedures of the Royal Society of Medicine 52:1031, 1959.

10. Burns, R.P.: Delayed onset of chloroquine retinopathy. The New England Journal of Medicine 275:693, 1966.

11. Scherbel, A., et al.: Ocular lesions in rheumatoid arthritis and related disorders with particular reference to retinopathy. The New England Journal of Medicine 273:360, 1965.

12. Mackenzie, A.H.: An appraisal of chloroquine. Arthritis and Rheumatism 13:280, 1970.

13. Hollander, J.L.: Calculated risk of arthritis treatment. American Journal of Medicine 62:1062, 1965.

14. Bothermich, H.O.: Coming catastrophe with chloroquine. Annals of Internal Medicine 61:1203, 1964.

15. Mainland, D. and Sutcliff, M.I.: Hydroxychloroquine sulfate in rheumatoid arthritis: A six-month double-blind trial. Bulletin on Rheumatic Diseases 13:207, 1962.

16. Popert, A.J., et al.: Chloroquine diphosphate in rheumatoid arthritis. Annals of Rheumatic Disease 20:18, 1961.

17. Rinehart, R.E., et al.: Chloroquine therapy in rheumatoid arthritis. Northwest Medicine 57:483, 1958.

18. Goldman, J.A. and Hess, E.V.: Treatment of rheumatoid arthritis. Bulletin on Rheumatic Diseases 21:609, 1970.

19. Saunders, T.S., et al.: Decrease in human hair color and feather pigment of fowl following chloroquine diphosphate. Journal of Investigational Dermatology 33:87, 1959.

20. Rynes, R.I., et al.: Ophthalmological safety of long-term hydroxychloroquine. Arthritis and Rheumatism 21:588, 1978.

21. Bernstein, H.N.: Chloroquine ocular toxicity. Survey of Ophthalmology 12:415, 1968.

CHAPTER 7: GOLD THERAPY

GOLD COMPOUNDS IN THE
TREATMENT OF RHEUMATOID ARTHRITIS

Gold, in use over 50 years, has withstood the test of time. Every few years a new class of rheumatologists decides that previous studies were inadequate, modifies the experimental design, and comes up with the same answer: Gold works.[1,2,3]

In the years 1971 to 1977, over 300 papers were published on gold.[6]

In 1890, Koch demonstrated that gold cyanide inhibited the tubercle bacillus in vitro. In 1927, Lande reported the successful use of gold thioglucose in rheumatoid arthritis, and Forestier, reasoning that rheumatoid arthritis and tuberculosis had certain similarities and that gold salt had been used successfully in treating tuberculosis, introduced gold therapy into the United States.[4]

Gold was greeted coldly in this country. In my internship (1938), the one man who dared to use gold was disdained. By 1948, when I started private practice, gold was still rarely used by many rheumatologists, largely because of its toxicity. The standard textbooks in arthritis at that time warned not to start gold therapy prior to obtaining the signed consent of the patient in the presence of two witnesses.[5] The major problem was that the prescribed dose of 100 mg of gold salt given for 10 injections carried a high incidence of serious toxicity and mortality for which there was no successful antidote.

The evolution of smaller doses lessened the frequency of severe reactions, and the eventual introduction of cortisone and BAL (British anti-lewisite) as antidotes added to the treating physician's sense of security.

Gold sodium thiomalate (Myochrysine) and aurothioglucose (Solganal) are the two gold preparations currently in use in the

United States. It is generally but not universally accepted that both compounds are equal as to efficacy and toxicity.[6,7]

Gold sodium thiomalate is a clear liquid and easily administered. Aurothioglucose is in an oil base which makes administration somewhat more difficult and introduces the injection of an oil along with the gold. My personal preference is for the gold thiomalate, except patients who develop nitronoid reactions to thiomalate (flushing-fainting) usually do not have these reactions with Aurothioglucose. An oral gold preparation, SKFD39162 (Auranofin), is currently being evaluated but is not available for general use.[8]

The current recommended schedule for the administration of gold consists of a 10 mg intramuscular injection of gold compound as a test dose. If no reaction occurs, a second test dose of 25 mg of gold compound is given one week later. If there are no side effects, a regular schedule of 50 mg once a week intramuscularly is started for 20 weeks for a total of 1,000 mg gold salt. If no significant improvement occurs, preference is to abandon the gold; however, a few physicians would advocate increasing the gold schedule.

If gold salt helps, then the patient should be maintained on gold for life. Stopping the gold will result in an exacerbation of the disease, and the patient seldom responds as well to the second course of gold. Maintenance therapy is accomplished by adhering to the 50 mg schedule but gradually increasing the time interval between injections. A common procedure is to shift to injections every two weeks for two to 20 weeks, then to every three weeks for three or four injections, and then to every fourth week. The patient is then continued on 50 mg of gold salt every fourth week for an indefinite period of time.[9]

The dosage of gold is empiric. Controlled studies have demonstrated increased toxicity and no benefit from large doses.[10] A dosage schedule of 25 mg a week of gold sodium thiomalate has proven as effective as 50 mg.[11]

Attempts have been made to individualize the gold dosage by monitoring the serum gold level,[12] but the difficulty in obtaining accurate serum gold levels makes this procedure impractical at this time for the average physician, and the method has not been universally successful.[11]

There is, then, a certain rationale to empiric individual variations in the gold salt dosage. As a general rule, use 50 mg of gold compound once a week for 20 doses and if successful go to a maintenance dosage schedule. But if the patient achieves a satisfactory remission before receiving the full 20-week course, shift at that time to a maintenance gold schedule to lessen the chances for toxicity. In a few susceptible individuals, a 25 mg weekly program can be successful.

The administration of gold should not be lightly undertaken, as the estimated current mortality is 0.4% or less. At one time the mortality approached 3 to 5%,[6] a higher mortality than occurs with many major surgical procedures.

Gold can affect almost any organ system. The most common side effect is dermatitis or stomatitis, but renal damage, bone marrow depression, eosinophilia, enterocolitis, peripheral neuritis, and alopecia[6] are the usual reactions. Reactions even more exotic and difficult to recognize, such as encephalopathy,[13] thrombocytopenia occurring late after the gold is discontinued,[14] or pulmonary fibrosis,[15,16] have also been reported.

Most gold reactions are minor. When they occur, gold should be temporarily discontinued and then resumed again on a regular or reduced dosage schedule after another initial test dose of 10 mg of gold compound. However, in case of bone marrow depression or thrombocytopenia, it is recommended that the drug not be resumed.

At each visit during which gold is administered, the patient should be questioned as to whether he has an itch, rash, sore mouth, metallic taste, diarrhea, or any unusual symptom. If any unusual symptom is present, the gold should be withheld until the symptoms clear. The laboratory should perform a complete blood count, an examination of the blood smear for adequate platelets, and a urinalysis at each visit and a platelet count at least once a month. Albuminuria, a low white blood count, inadequate platelets, a sudden drop in hemoglobin, and a rapid rise in sedimentation are all signals to withhold the gold until the problem is solved.

An occasional patient will complain of an exacerbation of the arthritis following gold injections. Many physicians encourage the patient to continue the gold in spite of this symptom. In my experience, however, exacerbation is usually a discouraging sign, and I do not persist if the symptoms repeat themselves with each gold injection.

Before starting gold, diagnosis should be firmly established. Gold should not be used in allergic individuals or in patients with systemic lupus erythematosus. Psoriasis is not a contraindication to gold, but other skin diseases or a history of eczema or allergy should be considered as a relative contraindication.

THE TREATMENT OF GOLD COMPLICATIONS

In spite of careful monitoring, gold complications do occur. The commonest complication is a dermatitis, usually accompanied by itching. The dermatitis may mimic almost any form of skin disease. Often the first sign of an impending dermatitis is a generalized itching, and if the patient complains of this symptom the gold should be temporarily withheld. Once a dermatitis develops, no matter how minute, the gold should be withheld until the dermatitis clears. If the dermatitis is disconcerting to the patient it usually can be treated with topical corticosteroids. In severe cases the short course of oral prednisone is necessary. This often offers prompt symptomatic relief. Once the dermatitis is over the patient can again be started on gold. The usual custom is to try a test dose of 10 mg, wait a week; try a second test dose of 25 mg and then go to the full dose of 50 mg. If the dermatitis develops with the second attempt of gold then it is useless to continue with the gold therapy. Persistence in gold therapy in the presence of a dermatitis can lead to a severe exfoliative dermatitis. In such severe cases the use of chelating agents such as BAL should be considered.

Stomatitis, which is not an unusual complication, can be so severe that the patient has difficulty in maintaining nutrition. In such cases a bland diet, local anesthetics such as Xylocaine gels may be tried, and in more severe cases oral corticosteroids. The development of a stomatitis is not a contraindication to a second trial of gold, but in my experience once a patient develops stomatitis it is very prone to recur if the gold is tried again.

Thrombocytopenia may occur early in the disease or even after therapy is discontinued. Occasionally it may not be recognized by the laboratory and may be first recognized by the patient as an idiopathic subcutaneous hemorrhage or nose bleed or genitourinary bleeding. The development of thrombocytopenia demands immediate cessation of therapy. From a laboratory point of view if the platelet count drops to 100,000 or less, gold therapy should be discontinued and not resumed. The patient developing a thrombocytopenia should be carefully evaluated to be certain that there are no other drugs that might be a factor. Any of these drugs that could be contributing to the thrombocytopenia should be immediately discontinued. The treatment of thrombocytopenia is variable. It seems to respond dramatically to large doses of prednisone, 40-100 mg daily maintained for at least a month and then slowly tapered, carefully monitoring the platelet count. If tapered too rapidly, there can be an exacerbation. In extreme cases chelating agents such as BAL or penicillamine may be used. During emergencies whole blood or platelet transfusion may be of value.

Leukopenia is not uncommon and must be watched for whenever the white blood cell count drops below 3,000. Then the gold should not be given. It is usually the granulocytes that are affected. If the leukopenia comes on unexpectedly and suddenly, the patient should be hospitalized for protective isolation. The treatment of leukopenia is empiric and poorly defined. It is uncertain whether the patient should be given whole blood or whether steroids help. It is well to involve a hematologist in such situations.

Aplastic anemia is a very serious complication with a high mortality. The development of this complication necessitates hospitalization and hematologic consultation, since the therapy at best is nonspecific and empiric and the prognosis is poor.

One of the more serious complications of gold therapy is of gold-induced nephrosis; this occurs if gold is given in spite of the development of proteinuria. The presence of protein in urine is a signal for discontinuing gold therapy. The urine should be checked for protein at each visit. A simple test with a dipstick as a screen procedure can be performed. Even if a trace of protein is present in the urine the gold should be withheld until protein is absent from the urine. If proteinuria persists and is progressive one must consider whether it is gold-induced or secondary to the disease. It is conceivable that the proteinuria may be due to amyloidosis or it may be that the original diagnosis was incorrect and the patient has systemic lupus erythematosus or scleroderma. In persistent proteinuria of any consequence a complete renal workup is indicated; this includes such studies as BUN, blood creatine, a creatinine clearance test, possibly an intravenous pyelogram and cystoscopic examination, and in some cases a renal biopsy may be indicated to establish a diagnosis.

Since gold toxicity may involve any organ system, particularly the lung, the gut, the liver, the eye, or the nervous system, any unusual manifestation of disease in these systems should be considered as possible gold toxicity until proven otherwise. The gold should be discontinued until the diagnosis is established. Alopecia, although a very rare complication of gold therapy because of its cosmetic problems, can be a difficult problem. In these circumstances the patient should be informed and should make the decision as to whether to continue gold and suffer the alopecia, or to stop the gold and consider other forms of therapy for the arthritis.

SUMMARY

Gold is an effective treatment for patients with rheumatoid arthritis and psoriatic arthritis. The usual dosage is two test doses; first 10 mg then 25 mg, followed by a weekly dose of 50 mg of gold compound intramuscularly once a week for 20 weeks, and then a reduction to a maintenance schedule of 50 mg every four weeks for life. The dosage of gold is empiric and smaller doses may be effective. Larger doses do not increase efficacy but do increase toxicity. The most common toxic reaction is dermatitis or albuminuria, but, as almost anything can occur, withhold the gold if any unusual symptoms develop. Do not persist with gold if results are doubtful.

Two forms of gold are available: thiomalate, which is water-soluble, and thiogluconate, which is in an oil base. The preferred form has never been definitely identified. The thiogluconate is less likely to cause nitronoid reactions but does introduce the oil as a foreign body, and its thicker solution is a little more difficult to administer.

REFERENCES

1. Empire Rheumatism Council: Gold therapy in rheumatoid arthritis. Annals of Rheumatic Disease 19:95-117, 1960.

2. Empire Rheumatism Council: Gold therapy in rheumatoid arthritis. Bulletin on Rheumatic Diseases 40:235-238, 1960.

3. The Cooperative Clinics of the ARA: A controlled trial of gold salt therapy in rheumatoid arthritis. Arthritis and Rheumatism 16:353, 1973.

4. Freyberg, R.H.: Gold Therapy for Rheumatoid Arthritis in Comroe's Arthritis, 5th ed. Lea and Febiger, Philadelphia, 1953.

5. Comroe, B.I.: Arthritis and Allied Conditions, 3rd ed. Lea and Febiger, Philadelphia, 1944.

6. Gohlieb, N.L.: Chrysotherapy. Bulletin on the Rheumatic Diseases 27:912-917, 1976-77.

7. Rothermich, N.O., et al.: Chrysotherapy: A prospective study. Arthritis and Rheumatism 19:1321-1327, 1976.

8. Finkelstein, A.E., et al.: Auranofin: New oral gold compound for the treatment of rheumatoid arthritis. Annals of Rheumatic Disease 35:251-257, 1976.

9. Smith, R.T., et al.: Increasing the effectiveness of gold therapy in rheumatoid arthritis. Journal of the American Medical Association 167:1197-1204, 1958.

10. Furst, D.E., et al.: A double-blind trial of high versus conventional dosages of gold salts for rheumatoid arthritis. Arthritis and Rheumatism 20:1473-1479, 1977.

11. Sharp, J.T., et al.: Comparison of the dosage schedules of gold salts in the treatment of rheumatoid arthritis. Arthritis and Rheumatism 20:1179-1187, 1977.

12. Lorber, A., et al.: Monitoring serum gold levels to improve chrysotherapy in rheumatoid arthritis. Annals of Rheumatic Disease 32:133-139, 1973.

13. McAuley, D.L.F., et al.: Gold encephalopathy. Journal of Neurology, Neurosurgery, and Psychiatry 40:1021-1022, 1977.

14. Stafford, B.T. and Crosby, W.H.: Late onset of gold-induced thrombocytopenia. Journal of the American Medical Association 239:50-51, 1978.

15. Scharf, J., et al.: Diffuse pulmonary injury associated with gold. Journal of the American Medical Association 237: 2410, 1977.

16. Winterbauer, R.H., et al.: Diffuse pulmonary injury associated with gold treatment. The New England Journal of Medicine 294:919-921, 1976.

CHAPTER 8:   PENICILLAMINE

"Penicillamine - will this young upstart replace gold?"

Penicillamine (Cuprimine) is a derivative of penicillin. It exists in three forms: D, DL, L. The D form, the least toxic, is the one used in clinical practice.

The chemical was initially found in 1953 in the urine of a patient with liver disease being treated with penicillin. At that time it was demonstrated that when given to animals it increased copper excretion and because of that it has been tried as a chelating agent in lead, mercury, and gold poisoning. It has been used successfully in Wilson's disease and cystinuria,[1] diseases which are ordinarily fatal.

In 1962, Jaffe demonstrated that intra-articular injection of D-penicillamine induced dissociation of the rheumatoid factor in synovial fluid but short-term oral therapy had no effect.[2] Long-term therapy using 2 grams a day orally resulted in clinical improvement.[3]

Jaffe's publications continued and in 1970 he reported favorably on 49 patients who had had long-term therapy.

In his initial work Jaffe used large initial doses, 2 to 4 grams daily, but the incidence of adverse effects was great and included a fatality from agranulocytosis.   Tolerance to the drug improved when Jaffe changed to a starting dose of 250 mg a day, increasing the dose 250 mg every two weeks until a maintenance dose of 1,500 mg a day was reached.[5]

In 1973, the British published a favorable report on efficacy in rheumatoid arthritis of D-penicillamine. The schedule used was Jaffe's step increments using two 250 mg capsules every two weeks for a total dosage of 3,000 mg. Toxicity was high but for those who were able to continue, the results were good.[6] This study legitimatized a popularly used drug in the United Kingdom.[5]

In this country the drug has recently been approved as therapy for rheumatoid arthritis. O'Brien warns that dosage schedules of 250 mg capsules increasing the dose every two weeks represents such a high risk that the ratio of benefits to risk may be totally unacceptable.[7]

Recently, there have been some suggestions that a lower dosage schedule might lessen toxicity and still might be efficacious.[8]

Jaffe now advocates a dosage schedule of "go low-go slow." Although the optimum dosage schedule still has not been resolved, Jaffe's current recommendation is to start with a 250 mg capsule a day and wait three months before increasing to 500 mg a day, and then wait another three months before going to 750 mg a day, and another three months before going to a maximum dose of 1 gram a day. A 125 mg capsule is now available and Jaffe suggests that reducing the dose 125 mg a day may eliminate undesirable side effects and maintain benefits. The duration of therapy has not been resolved but appears to be the minimum effective dose maintained indefinitely. Some clinicians suggest dropping the maintenance dose by 125 mg every three months. Some exacerbations may occur on this program but do not necessitate raising the dose as the flare may be self-limiting. If there are treatment failures at the end of four or five years, Jaffe recommends a six-month rest period and trying again.

Toxicity with the drug is a major problem and requires constant monitoring, according to Jaffe. The major side effects are:

1. Hematological - leukopenia and thrombocytopenia. Stop the drug if the WBC drops below $3,000/mm^3$ or the platelet count below $100,000/mm^3$ and do not rechallenge.

2. Renal proteinuria. If proteinuria persists and exceeds 2 grams a day, and does not drop with the reduction of dose, do not persist. A severe nephrotic syndrome can develop.

3. Autoimmune. Autoimmune diseases have been reported (Goodpasture's syndrome, myasthenia gravis, polymyositis, pemphigus, lupuslike disease, bronchiolitis).

4. Skin reactions. Pruritus and rash occur and may respond to lowered doses or antihistamines.

5. Drug fever is an indication for stopping therapy.

6. Stomatitis, if it persists, necessitates stopping the drug.

7. Loss of taste is common and usually disappears gradually. Elemental zinc 30-50 mg a day taken for a short period of time, but never along with the penicillamine, has been suggested as an antidote.

8. A benign enlargement of the breast has been reported.[9]

MY OPINION

Penicillamine is effective and may work when other drugs fail. It is toxic but Jaffe's "go low-go slow" regime may make the drug acceptable. The drug should be considered experimental, although now approved for therapy in cases resistant to older conventional therapy, and the patient should be advised of its experimental nature and toxicity. The patient should also be warned to discontinue the drug at once if any unusual symptoms or signs develop. The physician should see the patient at frequent intervals. At the onset of therapy, a complete blood count, platelet count, and urine analysis is performed and repeated every two weeks, but as time progresses the interval between laboratory tests may be increased.

The drug should not be used in pregnancy, and at this time there is no evidence that it is of value in other rheumatic diseases such as systemic sclerosis and vasculitis, but it is being tried experimentally.

SUMMARY

D-penicillamine threatens to replace gold as a drug of choice in the treatment of rheumatoid arthritis. It comes as a 125 mg and 250 mg capsule. Recent advice to start with a low dose of 250 mg daily and increase the dose 250 mg every three months to a maximum of 1 gm appears to have lessened toxicity but not lessened efficacy. The drug is toxic and must be carefully monitored, particularly for bone marrow depression, thrombocytopenia, and albuminuria.

REFERENCES

1. Meniot, A.G. and Huskison, E.C.: D-penicillamine. In: Rheumatoïd Arthritis Clinics in Rheumatic Diseases. W. B. Saunders Co., Philadelphia, 1975, p. 319.

2. Jaffe, I.A.: Intraarticular dissociation of the rheumatoid factor. Journal of Laboratory and Clinical Medicine 60:409, 1962.

3. Jaffe, I.A.: Comparison of the effects of plasmapheresis and penicillamine on the level of circulation rheumatoid factor. Annals of Rheumatic Disease 22:71, 1963.

4. Jaffe, I.A.: The treatment of rheumatoid arthritis and necrotizing vasculitis with penicillamine. Arthritis and Rheumatism 13:436, 1970.

5. Hill, H.F.: Treatment of rheumatoid arthritis with penicillamine. Seminars in Arthritis and Rheumatism 6:361, 1977.

6. Multicentre trial group: Controlled trial of D-penicillamine in severe rheumatoid arthritis. Lancet 1:275, 1973.

7. O'Brien, W.M.: Paper presented before the American Society of Clinical Pharmacology and Therapeutics. Atlanta, Ga., March 30, 1978.

8. Shiokawa, Y., et al.: Clinical evaluation of D-penicillamine by multicentre double-blind comparative study in chronic rheumatoid arthritis. Arthritis and Rheumatism 20:1464, 1977.

9. Jaffe, I.A.: D-penicillamine. Bulletin on the Rheumatic Diseases 28:948, 1977-78.

CHAPTER 9:   THE CORTICOSTEROIDS

"A Blessing and a Curse"

In 1949, Hench, Kendall, Slocumb, and Polly revolutionized rheumatology when they described the dramatic effects of cortisone in the treatment of rheumatoid arthritis.[1] As one of the era's leading rheumatologists, Hench for years had searched for an elusive "X" substance which would suppress rheumatoid arthritis. He was impressed by the fact that jaundice or pregnancy could induce a remission even in severe cases, and he was convinced that a physiological substance existed that could alter the course of the disease. While Hench, as a clinician, searched for the elusive "X" compound, biologic chemists such as Kendall[10] at the Mayo Clinic and Reichenstein in Switzerland were preparing extracts of the adrenal gland which they hoped would be of some benefit in Addison's disease (adrenal insufficiency). Hench tried one of these extracts named cortin but noted no effect in rheumatoid arthritis.   By 1935 it was recognized that adrenal cortical extracts contained a number of chemical compounds with varying physiological activity. These compounds were labeled A, B, E, and S. Compound E was eventually named cortisone by Hench and Kendall. As early as 1941, Kendall and Hench wanted to administer compound A, but a sufficient amount did not exist to treat even one rheumatic patient.   At that time, 3000 pounds of beef adrenal gland were required to produce 1 gram of compound A, and it was impossible to separate by biological means enough of these compounds for practical clinical use.   Chemical synthesis was attempted by Merck & Co., whose chemists finally synthesized enough compound A to test the material in a patient with Addison's disease.   Compound A proved a failure. The chemists persevered, however, and in 1948, Lewis H. Sarett, a Merck chemist, synthesized compound E, today's cortisone. Production of a few grams of compound E required bile from 40 oxen and nine months of synthesis. It was tested successfully in three patients with Addison's disease, but its production costs could not justify continued production. When

Hench asked Merck for a few grams of this precious substance to treat a patient with rheumatoid arthritis, a pitifully small amount existed in the entire world.[2]

The introduction of cortisone into clinical medicine exploded a bombshell. First and foremost, it legitimized the practice of rheumatology, and secondly, it stimulated hope that a successful treatment had been discovered, although from the onset Hench had described his work as a physiologic experiment and not a treatment.[3]

Cortisone does indeed produce dramatic results in inflammatory diseases. In adequate doses, all signs of inflammation disappear. Initially, when the drug was introduced, it was administered in large doses, 300 mg daily, and then slowly reduced in the hopes that the amazing remission would be sustained. It did not take long for the bad news to break. Not only was the remission not maintained, but often the exacerbation of the arthritis following the withdrawal of cortisone was worse than the original attack and even more distressing, the patient now had two diseases, rheumatoid arthritis and cortisone withdrawal effects.[5]

The corticosteroid derivatives from the adrenal gland are of two types physiologically. The glucorticosteroids primarily influence carbohydrate metabolism; the mineral corticosteroids affect salt retention. It is the glucocorticosteroids that exhibit an anti-inflammatory effect and hence are of concern in the treatment of rheumatic diseases.[8] Hydrocortisone replaced cortisone for clinical treatment when pharmaceutical chemists increased cortisone's potency without increasing its toxicity by modification of an OH radical. Hydrocortisone became the accepted standard, and the pharmaceutical companies raced to increase the anti-inflammatory effects and decrease the side effects. They succeeded in increasing the potency but not in eliminating the side effects. Some of these newer compounds had as much as 100 times the anti-inflammatory effect of hydrocortisone, but the toxicity, particularly salt retention, precluded many from clinical use. Today there exist at least 20 generic glucocorticosteroids in clinical use. A partial list of some of the best known follows:

1. Cortisone
2. Hydrocortisone
3. Betamethasone
4. Fluprednisolone
5. Meprednisone
6. Prednisolone

7. Prednisone
8. Triamcinolone

Betamethosone is 30 times as potent an anti-inflammatory agent
as hydrocortisone and has no salt retaining properties. Each of
the compounds varies in its half-life, anti-inflammatory potency,
and effect on mineral metabolism.[8,9] In different situations,
one compound may have some advantage over the other, but from
a practical point of view, when used in rheumatic diseases, most
rheumatologists have settled on prednisone as the standard. It
is readily available as a generic and hence less costly and is
available in both 1 and 5 mg tablets, making it easier to minutely
adjust dosage.

In the pituitary gland, adrenocorticotropic hormone, (ACTH),
stimulates the adrenal gland to produce excessive amounts of
cortisone-like (cortisol) hormones. The substance was originally isolated by Collip and associates in 1933,[11] and Hench in
his original trials ascribed the same therapeutic properties to
ACTH as he did to cortisone. The ACTH used by Hench was a
partially purified natural extract of animal pituitary glands. The
ACTH used now clinically is marketed in the form of depot preparations either in a gel or a zinc preparation. Because they provide therapeutically active blood levels of glucocorticoids for 24
to 48 hours following a single intramuscular injection, they have
achieved some popularity.[12] Shorter acting preparations of ACTH
are available. They are either biologic extracts or a synthetic
analogue, and are used primarily as diagnostic test material.
The synthetic ACTH is less likely to cause sensitivity reactions.

As a general rule, ACTH is not used as a therapeutic tool in
rheumatology because it must be given intramuscularly and has
been known to produce antigens which may cause serious or even
fatal reactions.[13] As a result, ACTH is seldom used in the treatment of chronic conditions. Some experts will use it for a short
"lift" in patients with a very active disease and in gout combined
with other anti-inflammatory agents. A few physicians have recommended it in place of prednisone as long-term therapy;[12] this
recommendation has not received general acceptance.

In prolonged use, the toxicity of the corticosteroids can be divided into three distinct components:

1. Side effect of the drug itself
2. Suppression of the pituitary adrenal axis
3. Reactivation of the initial disease process

Steroidal side effects are distressing because they are real and common. When we read about side effects of other drugs, we expect them to occur only in rare cases. The ratio of therapeutic benefit to toxicity is low. This is not true with chronic steroid use. Almost all patients develop suppression of the pituitary adrenal axis and are at increased risk during times of stress such as surgery, trauma, or infection. Most of the patients on long-term use will develop round face and obesity (women more likely than men). Many will develop peptic ulcer with perforation or bleeding or compression fractures of the vertebra.

The therapeutic principles are as follows:[14]

1. The appropriate dose is determined by trial and error.

2. A single dose, even a large one, is virtually without side effects.

3. A few days of corticosteroid in the absence of specific indications or excessive doses is unlikely to produce side effects, but its effects on the rheumatoid patient are so spectacular that its withdrawal may be psychologically impossible.

4. After prolonged use, the pituitary adrenal function may be suppressed for as long as nine months to a year. During this period and for an additional one to two years, patients need to be protected during stressful situations.[14]

5. As the corticosteroid therapy is prolonged, the incidence of side effects increases.

6. The drug is not curative. It is a palliative. It is probable that it does not alter the course of rheumatoid arthritis as a disease. Rather, it may even permit or hasten its progression due to the avoidance of rest and the overuse of damaged joints.

7. The abrupt withdrawal of steroids can lead to adrenal insufficiency and death.

The complications of long-term therapy can include:

1. Pituitary adrenal suppression
2. Fluid and electrolyte disturbance - sodium retention, potassium depletion.
3. Hyperglycemia and glycosuria
4. Increased susceptibility to infections

5. Peptic ulcers
6. Myopathy
7. Behavioral disturbances, including frank psychosis
8. Changes in physical appearance - moon face, humped shoulders (buffalo hump), and obesity
9. Supraclavicular fat pads
10. Skin ecchymosis, acne, hirsutism
11. Osteoporosis and vertebral fractures[15]
12. Cataracts

To lessen side effects, various regimens have been suggested such as alternate-day therapy and a single dose only in the morning.[16] Additional suggestions to lessen side effects have included the use of ulcer diets and antacids to prevent peptic ulcer formation, anabolic agents or sodium fluoride to counteract the osteoporosis, and in long-term therapy some experts do try these prophylactic measures.[17]

During stress or surgery the patient who has been on cortisone should be protected by excess corticosteroids. The following empiric regimen suggested by Hess and Goldman[18] has withstood the test of time:

Surgery day 1: Hydrocortisone IM at 6 AM and Solu-Medrol, 30 mg or Decadron, 6.5 mg every eight hours in IV fluid during surgery beginning prior to anesthesia. Hydrocortisone, 100 mg IV, should be available in case of signs of adrenal insufficiency, tachycardia, hypotension, or vascular collapse.

Day 2: Solu-Medrol 15 mg or Decadron 3 mg IM every eight hours

Day 3: Solu-Medrol 10 mg or Decadron 2 mg IM every eight hours

Day 4: Prednisone by mouth 15 mg in the morning, 10 mg in the afternoon

Day 5: Prednisone 10 mg twice a day

Day 6: Prednisone 10 mg in the morning, 5 mg in the afternoon.

Thereafter, each day decrease the dose until the patient is back on the maintenance dose. The use of synthetic corticosteroids avoids electrolyte problems.

In 1951, a microcrystalline form of hydrocortisone acetate was produced. It had the advantage over previous cortisone preparations that were injected intra-articularly. It was slowly absorbed and produced local anti-inflammatory effects without systemic effects. Hollander introduced the technique into clinical medicine.[19]

Since that time there have been various modifications of steroids for intra-articular use. Currently, the commonly available preparations are:

1. Hydrocortisone acetate: 25 to 50 mg per cc
2. Prednisone tertiary butyl acetate: 20 mg per cc
3. Triamcinolone hexacetonide: 5 and 20 mg per cc
4. Betamethasone acetate and sodium phosphate: 6 mg per cc
5. Methylprednisolone acetate: 20 and 40 mg per cc.[20]

Although there is a theoretical variation in the potency of the various preparations, the dosage is usually prescribed in cc of solution and depends on the size of the joint. Thus, in the knee, 1 to 2 cc of solution are commonly injected while only 0.1 cc may be injected in the metatarsal phalangeal joint.

In general, intra-articular corticosteroids will reduce inflammation in an inflamed joint, but their effects are transitory. Whether the newer preparations prolong the beneficial effects is uncertain. Intra-articular steroids are used in rheumatoid and degenerative joints. In about one percent of the cases the injection may result in an exacerbation of the inflammation.[21] The injection must be accomplished under aseptic technique, as the greatest danger is the introduction of an infection, a rare but serious complication. A septic arthritis is a contraindication to steroid injection. Any joint can be injected. The smaller the joint, the smaller the volume of injected material. Injection of the hip, once common, is now generally avoided, as its depth necessitates a difficult technical approach and the material is often deposited outside of the joint instead of in the joint.

The occasional injection of an acute joint is worthwhile, but repeated long-term injection is inadvisable because of the dangers of permitting overuse, thus damaging a diseased joint, and of introducing an infection. I currently inject fewer joints than in the past, because with total joint replacement becoming increasingly popular, the danger of introducing a latent infection with subsequent rejection of the artificial joint is real.

The dosage of cortisone to be used is discussed in the chapters on the individual diseases.

SUMMARY

Nothing equals the dramatic effect of the corticosteroids in the rheumatic diseases.

The physician therefore has at his disposal a dramatic weapon. If he chose to treat every patient with rheumatic complaints with corticosteroids and ignore the diagnoses completely, the results would be dramatic and his wonders would be extolled for all to hear. His patients would shout with joy that they had been to lesser physicians who performed expensive tests, and when all was said and done had nothing to offer but aspirin or more expensive substitutes, while the physician who used steroids performed miracles. His waiting room would be full and the press would proclaim his glory and he could laugh all the way to the bank. It has been done. The problem is that although steroids offer dramatic relief, and although there are certain and specific indications for their use, their indiscriminate use may actually produce more harm than good. In the treatment of rheumatoid arthritis, they certainly do not alter the course of the disease and in subsequent years, the relief that they have offered will have deteriorated and the patient will now be faced with two diseases instead of one. The rheumatoid arthritis will have progressed and the patient will now have to deal with the problems of cortisone toxicity and withdrawal.

Before beginning use of steroids, the following points should be considered:

1. A specific diagnosis must be established, since one is embarking on the use of a toxic drug.

2. The initial dosage should be appropriate to the clinical situation. Thus, in treating rheumatoid arthritis, one would start with a very low dosage, 2 to 3 mg, and build up slowly not to exceed 10 mg in 24 hours. In treating a severe complication of systemic lupus or lupus crisis, one might start with a minimum of 60 mg in a 24-hour period.

3. Steroids cause an increased excretion of sodium and potassium. When they are to be administered in large doses for long periods of time, blood electrolytes and blood glucose should be monitored.

4. Because of the natural rhythm of the pituitary adrenal axis, steroids are less likely to cause side effects if administered only once a day, preferably in the morning, as this causes

the least disturbance of the normal rhythm of the axis. Alternate-day therapy is even better in that it is less likely to cause side effects. However, alternate-day therapy is seldom effective in inflammatory rheumatic diseases, because the day the steroids are withheld the patient becomes much worse. Alternate-day therapy is practical only when there is very good control of the inflammatory process.

5. If alternate-day therapy is attempted, there is no point in using a long-acting steroid, because its effect flows over into the second day. The easiest practical short-acting steroid to use is prednisone with a half-life of only 60 minutes, as compared to triamcinolone with a half-life of 300 minutes.

6. Long-term steroid therapy may lead to serious eye problems such as cataract or increased intraocular tension. It is therefore advisable to get a baseline eye examination before starting long-term steroid therapy.

7. Steroid therapy, particularly in large doses for a long period of time, makes the patient more vulnerable to infections because it suppresses the immune protective system. Therefore, if the patient deteriorates while on steroid therapy, instead of increasing the steroid dosage, consider the possibility of a suppressed infection to be a complicating factor.

8. Large-dose and long-term steroids may actually mimic the disease being treated. Steroids may induce myalgia, arthralgia, hypertension, edema, and proteinuria. All these are manifestations of systemic rheumatic diseases. It is easy to make the error that the patient is deteriorating because of progression of the disease, whereas the deterioration may in actuality be steroid related: iatrogenic produced.[22,23,24]

9. The patient should be advised to carry information on his person that he is on steroids.

10. Do not forget supplemental steroid dosage when stress occurs. Even stress as minor as a tooth extraction should be covered.

The corticosteroids have the following pharmacologic and potentially undesirable effects:

1. They influence carbohydrate metabolism, resulting in a glycosuria and a steroid diabetes. This diabetes is usually insulin-resistant and without ketosis or acidosis.

2. They cause a negative nitrogen balance and a depletion of body protein stores with muscle wasting.

3. They cause a redistribution of fat with characteristic changes such as the buffalo hump and the round face.

4. They influence electrolyte and water metabolism, causing sodium retention with the resulting increased body fluid and secondary edema. In susceptible patients, this may lead to congestive heart failure. A hypokalemic alkalosis occurs and can be treated with potassium salts.

5. They suppress secretions of the pituitary gland resulting in atrophy of the adrenal glands and particular susceptibility to stress. In addition, hirsutism and occasional alterations in menstrual function can result in women.

6. They alter the inflammatory response and suppress the inflammatory reaction, possibly resulting in perforation of a peptic ulcer or spread of an infection.

7. They act as an anti-inflammatory agent and are said to suppress the mechanisms of tissue injury.

8. Osteoporosis may occur as the result of increased calcium removal from the bone.

9. They can produce lymphocytosis and on occasion a leukemoid reaction.

10. Gastric or duodenal ulcers may follow.

11. Hypervolemia, edema, and congestive failure can result from high doses.

12. Subcutaneous hemorrhages and acne result.

13. The central nervous system can be affected with psychoses, seizures, and psychologic changes and insomnia.

REFERENCES

1. Hench, P.S., et al.: The effect of a hormone of the adrenal cortex (17-Hydroxy-11-dehydrocortisone: Compound E) and

a pituitary adrenocorticotropic hormone on rheumatoid arthritis: Preliminary report. Proceedings of the Staff of the Mayo Clinic 24:181-197, 1949.

2. Hench, P.S.: A reminiscence of certain events before, during, and after the discovery of cortisone. Minnesota Medicine 36:705-710, 1953.

3. Hench, P.S., et al.: Effects of cortisone acetate and pituitary ACTH on rheumatoid arthritis, rheumatic fever, and certain other conditions: A study in clinical physiology. Archives of Internal Medicine 85:545, 1950.

4. Sarett, L.H., et al.: The effects of structural alteration on the anti-inflammatory properties of hydrocortisone. Progress in Drug Research 5:11-153, 1963.

5. Bernsten, C.A. and Freyberg, R.H.: Evaluation of the status of patients with rheumatoid arthritis after five or more years of corticosteroid therapy. Bulletin of Rheumatic Diseases 12:261-262, 1961.

6. Polley, H.F.: Evaluation of steroids and their value in control of rheumatic diseases. Mayo Clinic Proceedings 45:1-12, 1970.

7. Boland, E.W.: Antirheumatic potency of chemically modified adrenocortical steroids. American Journal of Medicine 3:581, 1961.

8. Dhehy, R.G., et al.: Pharmacology and Chemistry of Adrenal Steroids in Steroid Therapy. Azarnoff, D.L., (ed.), W.B. Saunders Co., Philadelphia, 1975, pp. 1-14.

9. Rose, L.I. and Saccar, C.: Choosing corticosteroid prerequisites. American Journal of Family Practice 17:198-204, 1978.

10. Mesou, H.L., et al.: The chemistry of crystalline gallstones isolated from the suprarenal gland. Journal of Biological Chemistry 114:613-631, 1936.

11. Collip, J.B., et al.: The adrenotropic hormone of the anterior pituitary lobe. Lancet 2:347-348, 1933.

12. Jasni, M.K.: The importance of ACTH and glucocorticoids. In: Rheumatic Arthritis Clinics in Rheumatic Diseases. W.B. Saunders Co., Philadelphia, 1975, p. 335.

13. Gloss, D. and Poly, J.R.: Development of antibodies during long-term therapy with corticotrophics in rheumatoid arthritis. American Journal of Rheumatologic Disease 30: 589-593, 1971.

14. Graber, A.L., et al.: Natural history of pituitary-adrenal recovery following long-term suppression with corticosteroids. Journal of Clinical Endocrinology and Metabolism 25:1-16, 1965.

15. Goodman, L.S. and Gilman, A.: The Pharmacological Basis of Therapeutics, 5th ed., Haynes, R.D. and Turner, J., (eds.), Macmillan Publishing Co., New York, 1975, pp. 1472-1506.

16. Horter, J.G., et al.: Studies on intermittent corticosteroid dosage regimen. New England Journal of Medicine 269:591-596, 1963.

17. Dujoune, C.A. and Azarnoff, D.L.: Clinical complications of corticosteroid therapy. In: Steroid Therapy, Azarnoff, D.L. (ed.), W.B. Saunders Co., Philadelphia, 1973.

18. Hess, E.V. and Goldman, J.A.: Corticosteroids and corticotropin. In: Therapy of Rheumatoid Arthritis and Allied Conditions, 8th Ed., Hollander, J.L. (ed.), Lea and Febiger, Philadelphia, 1972, pp. 495-516.

19. Hollander, J.L.: The local effects of compound F (hydrocortisone) injected into joints. Bulletin on Rheumatic Diseases 2:21, 1951.

20. Gifford, R.H.: Corticosteroid therapy for rheumatoid arthritis. In: Steroid Therapy, Azarnoff, D. L. (ed.), W.B. Saunders Co., Philadelphia, 1973, pp. 78-95.

21. McCarty, D.J. and Hogan, J.M.: Inflammatory reaction after intrasynovial injection of microcystalline adrenocorticosteroid esters. Arthritis and Rheumatism 7:359, 1965.

22. Hardin, J.C., Jr.: Steroid-induced morbidity mimicking active systemic lupus erythematosus. Annals of Internal Medicine 78:558, 1973.

23. Fauci, A.S., et al.: Glucocorticosteroid therapy: Mechanisms of action and clinical considerations. Annals of Internal Medicine 84:304, 1976.

24. Aagaard, G.N.: Drug spotlight on steroid therapy. Annals of Internal Medicine 84:551, 1976.

CHAPTER 10: IMMUNOSUPPRESSIVE DRUGS

> "The Devil must be exorcised. A bad disease
> requires a powerful drug."

These drugs were originally introduced as a treatment for cancer. Fosdick's reports of the successful use of cyclophosphamide (Cytoxan) and at the same time the development of the concept of "autoimmune disease" associated with abnormally functioning lymphocytes led to the popularization of the use of these drugs in inflammatory arthritis.[1,2]

The compounds currently in popular use in the United States are cyclophosphamide (Cytoxan), azathioprine (Imuran), chlorambucil (Leukeran), and methotrexate.

These drugs do not all act in the same way. Cyclophosphamide and chlorambucil belong to a class of drugs called alkylating agents. Alkylating agents kill cells during all phases of the cell cycle. Azathioprine belongs to a group of agents known as antimetabolites; these interfere with DNA synthesis, thus destroying rapidly dividing cells. Methotrexate belongs to a group which interferes with folic acid metabolism which is essential for DNA formation and therefore is essential for cell metabolism.[3]

These drugs are not "approved"* for the treatment of rheumatic diseases, nor have they been subjected to long-term evaluation, but there is a general consensus among rheumatologists that they are effective in rheumatoid arthritis, especially cyclophosphamide.[4] Their effectiveness in other diseases such as systemic lupus is questionable.[5,6] Because of cyclophosphamide's high toxicity, the other drugs have been used, and, in an attempt to lessen toxicity, decreasing doses have been tried.[4,7,8] In my opinion, none of the other drugs is as effective as cyclosphosphamide, nor is a smaller dose regimen as good as the full dose.[9,10]

*Methotrexate is approved for use in severe psoriatic arthritis.

All of these drugs have serious, fatal, irreversible side effects. All of them can cause bone marrow depression; all of them, by suppressing the immune system, open the patient to the hazard of increased susceptibility to infection. Herpes zoster, for example, is usually a benign disease in most people, but in an immune suppressed patient it may become systemic and fatal. On a theoretical basis and from experience gained in the immune suppressed transplant patients, there is evidence of an increased incidence of malignancy, especially with the use of cyclophosphamide.[11-15] All of these drugs can cause gastrointestinal upsets, and, in addition, some of these drugs have side effects peculiar to themselves individually. These side effects are discussed with the separate drugs. Dosage, however, is still an uncharted area. The basic principle followed has been to use the smallest dose possible to obtain a therapeutic effect. With cyclophosphamide, the margin between efficacy and toxicity has been thin.

In my opinion, these drugs have a very limited place in the treatment of rheumatoid arthritis; however, it is true that occasionally they work when all else has failed. The rheumatologists, therefore, must be acquainted with them to use in desperate situations. The physician and the patient must be aware of the risks involved.

CYCLOPHOSPHAMIDE

I have seen the disappearance of bone erosions and remissions with this drug superior in my experience to anything I have seen with any other drug. Unfortunately, its toxicity almost precludes its use. In addition to the previously mentioned side effects, it can produce an alopecia, a nonreversible hemorrhagic cystitis, and suppression of gonadal function. The incidence of these side effects is high.[8,11,12]

The general impression is that cyclophosphamide, to be effective, has to produce a leukopenia between 2,500 to 4,000 WBCs per ml. The suggested usual dose is 50 mg daily, increasing by 50 mg every four weeks until a maximum daily dose of 150 to 250 mg is reached (1.5 to 2.0 mg/kg), assuming that the patient tolerates it. In one study, 90% of the patients receiving the drug had side effects.[4]

CHLORAMBUCIL

The incidence of side effects has led to a trial of chlorambucil which theoretically acts in the same manner as Cytoxan. It appears to be less toxic but also less potent.[13,14,15]

The usual recommended dose is 4 to 8 mg daily until leukopenia is reached and then a minimum maintenance dose is followed.

AZATHIOPRINE

This drug is the current darling of those favoring immunosuppressive therapy; it is less toxic than cyclophosphamide and better tolerated. The suggested dose is 2 to 3 mg per kilogram per day, dropping to a maintenance dose of 1.5 mg per kilogram daily when improvement occurs. Leukopenia does not have to occur for the drug to be effective. It is probably not as effective as cyclophosphamide but less toxic.[16-19] Reversible chromosomal damage occurs in patients on cyclophosphamide or azathioprine.[20] Patients on azathioprine have had successful pregnancies but the risks should be considered.[21]

METHOTREXATE

This drug is used by some. It is given orally or intramuscularly in a dose of 25 to 37.5 mg once a week (0.5 to 1 mg/kg). It has been reported to be effective in psoriatic arthritis, dermatomyositis, and rheumatoid arthritis. Methotrexate may induce hair loss, cause oral ulcers, promote teratogenesis, cause hepatitis and cirrhosis of the liver. The Food and Drug Administration has given approval for the use of methotrexate in severe cases of psoriasis with arthropathic complications.[22,23]

SUMMARY

Do not consider the immunosuppressives unless more conservative measures have been tried.

Cyclophosphamide in a dosage of 150 to 200 mg daily is the most effective and the most toxic.

Azathioprine, 2 to 3 mg/kg or less in selected cases is almost as effective as cyclophosphamide and less toxic.

Chlorambucil is less toxic than the other drugs in its class. The usual dosage is 4 to 8 mg daily. It probably is the least effective.

Methotrexate is given once a week 25 to 37.5 mg (lesser doses may be effective). It can be given orally but is usually given intramuscularly, and it may be effective in severe psoriatic arthritis but its propensity to alopecia is a limiting factor, particularly in women, and the problem of severe fatal liver disease is a constant hazard. A liver biopsy should be done prior to treatment and at yearly intervals.

The use of these drugs requires experience, patient consent, and constant laboratory monitoring. The bone marrow suppression is a particularly serious problem. Methotrexate given parenterally produces its major leukopenic response on the third to fourth day after administration of the drug with a rapid recovery thereafter. The drug should be withheld if leukopenia persists before the next weekly dose. Cyclophosphamide at the recommended dosage level produces its major bone marrow depression in 10 to 14 days. Azathioprine produces its bone marrow depression in three to six weeks.[13] It is wise to do urine analysis, weekly blood and platelet counts until one gets the "feel" of the drugs. Do not expect a clinical result with these drugs in less than 30 to 90 days. If a good therapeutic response is obtained, maintenance therapy must be carried on indefinitely.[24-28]

REFERENCES

1. Fosdick, W.M., et al.: Cytotoxin therapy in rheumatoid arthritis. Medical Clinics of North America 52:747, 1968.

2. Fosdick, W.M., et al.: Long-term cyclophosphamide therapy in rheumatoid arthritis. Arthritis and Rheumatism 11: 151, 1968.

3. AMA Department of Drugs: Antineoplastic drugs. AMA Drug Evaluation, 3rd Ed., AMA Dept. of Drugs, P.S.G. Publishing Co., Littleton, 1977, p. 1107.

4. American Rheumatism Association Cooperating Clinics Committee: A controlled trial of cyclophosphamide in rheumatoid arthritis. The New England Journal of Medicine 283: 833, 1970.

5. Roghfield, J.F.: Immunosuppressive therapy in lupus erythematosus. Annals of Internal Medicine 76:619, 1972.

6. Decker, J.L., et al.: Cyclophosphamide or azathioprine in lupus glomerulonephritis. Annals of Internal Medicine 83: 606, 1975.

7. Urowitz, M.B., et al.: Azathioprine in rheumatoid arthritis: A double-blind cross-over study comparing full dose to half dose. Journal of Rheumatism 1:274, 1974.

8. Currey, H.L.F., et al.: Comparison of azathioprine, cyclophosphamide and gold in the treatment of rheumatoid arthritis. British Medical Journal 3:764, 1974.

9. Hurd, E.R. and Ziff, M.: Parameters of improvement in patients with rheumatoid arthritis treated with cyclophosphamide. Arthritis and Rheumatism 17:72, 1974.

10. Lidsky, M.D., et al.: Double-blind study of cyclophosphamide in rheumatoid arthritis. Arthritis and Rheumatism 16:148, 1973.

11. Aptekar, R.G., et al.: Bladder toxicity with chronic and cyclophosphamide therapy in now malignant disease. Arthritis and Rheumatism 16:461, 1975.

12. Fairley, K.F., et al.: Sterility and testicular atrophy related to cyclophosphamide treatment. Lancet 1:568-569, 1972.

13. Denman, E.J., et al.: Failure of cytotoxin drugs to suppress immune responsiveness of patients with rheumatoid arthritis. Annals of Rheumatic Disease 29:220-231, 1970.

14. Kahn, M., et al.: Immunosuppressive drugs in the management of malignant and severe rheumatoid arthritis. Procedures of the Royal Society of Medicine 60:130-133, 1967.

15. Santos, G.U.: Immunosuppressive drugs. I. Federation Proceedings 26:907-913, 1967.

16. Urowitz, M.B., et al.: Azathioprine treatment of rheumatoid arthritis: A double-blind cross-over study. Arthritis and Rheumatism 14:411-418, 1971.

17. Levy, J., et al.: A double-blind controlled evaluation of azathioprine in the treatment of rheumatoid and psoriatic arthritis. Arthritis and Rheumatism 15:116-117, 1972.

18. Mason, M., et al.: Azathioprine in rheumatoid arthritis. British Medical Journal 1:420, 1969.

19. Hunter, T., et al.: Azathioprine in rheumatoid arthritis. Arthritis and Rheumatism 18:15-20, 1975.

20. Tolchin, S.F., et al.: Chromosomal abnormalities from cyclophosphamide therapy in rheumatoid arthritis and progressive systemic sclerosis. Arthritis and Rheumatism 17 (4):375-382, 1974.

54/ Immunosuppressive Drugs

21. Ginzler, E., et al.: Long-term maintenance therapy with
    azathioprine in systemic lupus erythematosus. Arthritis
    and Rheumatism 18:27-34, 1975.

22. Ehrlich, G.E.: Chapter 44. Remittive Pharmaceutical
    Agents. In: Rheumatic Diseases. Katz, W. (ed.), J.B.
    Lippincott Co., Philadelphia, 1977, p. 67.

23. Poduraiel, B.A., et al.: Liver injury associated with meth-
    otrexate therapy for psoriasis. Mayo Clinic Proceedings
    48:787, 1973.

24. Kaplan, S.R. and Calabresi, P.: Immunosuppressive agents.
    The New England Journal of Medicine 289:952, 1973.

25. Steinberg, A.D., et al.: Cytotoxic drugs in treatment of
    nonmalignant diseases. Annals of Internal Medicine 78:619,
    1972.

26. Decker, J.L.: Toxicity of immunosuppressive drugs in
    man. Arthritis and Rheumatism 16:89, 1973.

27. Love, R.R. and Laura, J.M.: Myelomonocytic leukemia
    following cyclophosphamide therapy of rheumatoid disease.
    Annals of Rheumatic Disease 34:534, 1975.

28. Wall, R.L. and Clausen, K.P.: Carcinoma of the urinary
    bladder in patients receiving cyclophosphamide. The New
    England Journal of Medicine 293:271, 1975.

Part Two: THE DISEASES

CHAPTER 1: GOUT

> "Gentlemen, learn gout and all of its manifesta-
> tions. Your colleagues will often miss the diag-
> nosis. When you start practice, you will make
> the diagnosis and be an instant success."

> Philip Hench

Gout is among man's oldest and most painful diseases. One physician who suffered from the disease wrote: "Screw up the vises
tight as possible and you have rheumatism. Give them another
turn and you have gout." Another victim wrote: "If you want to
know what it feels like, take your eyeballs out of their sockets
and walk upon them." In 1932, a book review in the British
Journal of Medicine 1:153, implied that gout was almost an ex-
tinct disease. The disease was far from obliterated; rather, the
profession had decided not to recognize such a perverse antago-
nist. In actual fact, it had been estimated that in a general rheumatology clinic, at least five percent of the patients will have
gout. Berton Roueche, a medical writer describing the disease
in "The New Yorker," has called gout "a perverse, ungrateful,
maleficent malady."

Any acute, sudden, painful monoarticular arthritis in the male
should be considered gout until proven otherwise. In the classic case, the initial attack is an acute monoarticular arthritis
involving one of the peripheral joints, often the toe. The pain is
intolerable. On examination the joint is distended, inflamed,
and may suggest a cellulitis. Even if the disease is not diagnosed within a few weeks of onset, the arthritis will completely
subside and the patient will appear to completely recover. After
a period of time, months or years, another acute, severe attack
will occur and again, if undiagnosed, will resolve spontaneously.
However, the patient will continue to have recurrent attacks of
acute, painful monoarticular arthritis with complete subsidence
of signs and symptoms between attacks. As time progresses,
the interval between attacks will become shorter, and multiple
joints will become involved. Ultimately if untreated, the disease
becomes chronic and may even resemble rheumatoid arthritis.

It has long been known that the disease is associated with a hyperuricemia. Since uric acid is relatively insoluble, it precipitates into the joints, the kidneys, and the other tissues. In the joints, it is engulfed by lymphocytes, and the destruction of these lymphocytes and the release of toxins may precipitate acute attacks of monoarticular arthritis. Deposited in the kidneys, uric acid can form renal stones and can obstruct kidney function, resulting in gouty nephritis. Deposits of uric acid in the skin, particularly in the ears or over the elbows, are known as tophi, which may ulcerate and discharge.

The hyperuricemia in man is due to either an increased production of uric acid by the body or a decreased excretion of uric acid by the kidneys, or by a combination of both.[2] The diuretic agents used in the treatment of hypertension may cause hyperuricemia,[3] but surprisingly few hypertensive patients develop gouty arthritis.[4] Diagnosis of gout depends on the classic history, the demonstration of tophi, an elevated serum uric acid, and a good therapeutic response to colchicine. Recent studies have suggested that these findings are not as specific as once was thought. Hyperuricemia will eventually manifest itself in 98 percent of all patients with gout, but it may well be normal during the initial attacks.[5] Generations of medical students have been taught that the therapeutic response to colchicine is specific for gout but, alas, it now appears to be nonspecific and equally effective in pseudogout.[6] Diagnosis is best made either by examination of the chalky tophus discharge which can be easily picked up with a small needle, placed on a drop of saline on a slide, and examined under the standard microscope for needle-like uric acid crystals, or, optimally, by aspirating the joint fluid and examining the fluid under polarized light microscopy to distinguish between the needle-like uric acid crystals of gout and the long rectangular calcium pyrophosphate crystals of pseudogout.[7]

In treating gout there are two distinct problems: treating the acute severe attack of pain (the arthritis) and treating the hyperuricemia to prevent future attacks and complications. Separate the therapy! Do not treat the hyperuricemia during the acute attack! Acute attacks are thought to be due to movement of the uric acid; treating the hyperuricemia may aggravate or precipitate an acute attack of arthritis.

There are multiple options for the treatment of acute pain. The means selected depends on the circumstances and the experience of the physician. The traditional treatment is colchicine. Colchicine has been used since the days of the ancient Greeks. It is derived from the bulb of the autumn crocus and, until modern times, was prepared as a tincture or a wine. It is presently available as a purified 0.6 mg tablet. The treatment of an acute attack is two tablets (0.6 mg each) at once and one tablet every two hours until the acute pain is relieved or diarrhea occurs. The necessary dosage varies from patient to patient, but in the average patient, the usual dose is 8 to 12 tablets. Once this dose is established, it is supposed to be fixed for life. The use of narcotics during the hours it takes for the colchicine to be effective is acceptable. The advantage of using colchicine is its long established tradition of safety. The disadvantages are the time it takes to get relief (12 to 24 hours) and the resulting diarrhea. The other advantage that used to be claimed for colchicine was that it was specific for gout and therefore could be used as a diagnostic tool; this advantage has disappeared with the demonstration that colchicine's action may be nonspecific and may help other forms of arthritis.[6] Colchicine is available in solution for intravenous use. The usual dosage is up to 3 mg intravenously. Used in this way, a more rapid therapeutic response is attained and the diarrhea is averted. The disadvantage is that the material is very sclerosing and, if injected outside of the vein, can be extremely painful. Therefore, it must be given very carefully and is probably best given as a "piggyback" injection on a previously running intravenous solution.

A second alternative method is phenylbutazone, 100 mg tablet, two tablets four times a day taken with food or milk for four doses and then one tablet four times a day until the patient is totally symptom-free. Indomethacin, 50 mg four times a day, is as effective as phenylbutazone. Both have the disadvantage of possibly activating a peptic ulcer. Phenylbutazone may theoretically cause an agranulocytosis (1 in 50,000 cases), and indomethacin may cause headaches and mental confusion. Both, however, are very satisfactory ways of treating an acute attack of gouty arthritis and are commonly used. The advantages of their use is prompt relief with minimal side effects. Naproxen, ibuprofen, fenoprofen and sulindac, used in their usual doses, have all been reported to be effective in gout. I have had no personal experience in their use in this situation. If they prove to be rapidly effective, they would have the advantage of being less toxic, at least as we evaluate them today. However, it is my impression from reading the reports of their successful use that it takes longer to achieve pain relief with these drugs that it does with phenylbutazone or indomethacin.[8,9,10]

In the past, cortisone or ACTH has been recommended as a quick method of relieving an acute attack of gouty arthritis. The drawback of the method was that as soon as the steroid was withdrawn, the patient would exacerbate with an even worse attack. Accordingly, it was suggested that the cortisone or ACTH be combined with another drug, such as phenylbutazone, indomethacin, or colchicine. Although this is an extremely effective and rapid way for controlling the acute attack of gouty arthritis, I strongly recommend against it. One problem is that any drug combination increases the risk of toxicity, but the worst problem is that this treatment often results in exacerbation of the arthritis upon withdrawal of the steroid. I have seen a few cases where a simple acute attack of gouty arthritis thus treated has been converted into a chronic arthritis and then mistreated as a case of rheumatoid arthritis.

Only after the subsidence of the acute attack should the treatment of hyperuricemia be considered. The treatment of hyperuricemia may precipitate another attack of gout. It is therefore prudent at this point to start the patient on prophylactic colchicine. There is considerable clinical experience to support the concept that colchicine, taken in a dosage of one or two tablets (0.6 mg) daily for an indefinite period of time, is relatively safe. The patient should be advised to reduce the dose if any G.I. distress occurs and to increase the dose by one or two tablets for a short period of time if he feels an impending attack. It is usual to leave the patient on the colchicine until he has been symptom-free of any acute attack of gouty arthritis for at least one year. 1, 12

After the patient has been symptom-free for at least a month, treatment of the hyperuricemia should begin. The aim of this treatment is to lower the serum uric acid so that it is not precipitated in the joints or the tissues and to prevent future attacks of arthritis. The treatment today should be almost 100 percent effective. There are three drugs in general use today which effectively lower the body's uric acid pool: probenecid (Benemid), sulfinpyrazone (Anturane), and allopurinol (Zyloprim). Probenecid and sulfinpyrazone work by increasing the uric acid excretion through the kidney. 14, 15, 16 Since these drugs function by causing an increased amount of uric acid in the urine, there is danger of a uric acid stone forming in the kidney with their use. Therefore, they should not be prescribed in patients with a history of uric acid stones. A recently conceived technique is to check the patient's 24-hour urine uric acid excretion; if this exceeds one gram, classify the patient as a hypersecretor of uric acid and do not overload the kidneys with probenecid or sulfinpyrazone. Therapy with uricosuric agents should be started with a low dose, and the patient should be advised to drink enough fluids to maintain an adequate urine flow. Alkalization of the urine with potassium citrate is occasionally advised, but most clinicians content themselves with starting with low doses and maintaining an adequate urine flow to prevent the formation of uric acid stones. The preferred drug is probenecid. This is available as a 1/2-gram tablet, given in four divided doses to total 2 to 3 grams daily. Probenecid is the initial drug of choice, because it has stood the test of time and is relatively nontoxic. If it does not work, then sulfinpyrazone is substituted. This comes as a 100 mg tablet and is given 100 mg twice a day up to 100 mg four times a day. Since this drug is a derivative of phenylbutazone, it carries the onus of possibly causing an agranulocytosis, but this is an extremely rare occurrence. A patient taking a uricosuric agent should be advised to avoid other drugs, particularly aspirin, as these interfere with the uric acid excretion.

Allopurinol is a far superior uricosuric agent than the two pre- viously discussed drugs and acts in an entirely different manner. Purine nucleotides in normal human metabolism are broken down by a series of oxidation reactions to uric acid which is excreted in the urine. Allopurinol interferes with the xanthine oxidase en- zyme and prevents the formation of uric acid. Therefore, the end product of purine nucleotide metabolism when allopurinol is used is xanthine. This is much more soluble than uric acid and is readily excreted by the kidneys, thus effectively lowering the body's uric acid pool.[16] Allopurinol is not used as the initial drug of choice because it was not introduced into clinical medi- cine until 1962 and thus has not stood the test of time. In addi- tion, several adverse effects have been reported from its wide- spread use. The mild side effects include gastrointestinal dis- tress, diarrhea, headaches, pleuritis, fever, and maculopapu- lar rash; these subside promptly after withdrawal of the drug. There have been reports, however, of more serious and fatal reactions, such as agranulocytosis, exfoliative dermatitis, acute vasculitis, and hepatotoxicity.[17,18] Allopurinol is usually given in a single dose. It comes as a 100 or 300 mg tablet; the ordi- nary dose is 200 to 400 mg daily. However, doses as high as 1,000 mg daily have been utilized in nonresponders. In resist- ant cases, allopurinol may be combined with probenecid or sul- finpyrazone. Allopurinol is preferred where there is impaired renal function or poor response to other drugs. Actually, aside from its toxicity, allopurinol is by far the most effective of all the uricosuric agents. Tophi of long duration will disappear with allopurinol. The allopurinol may be so effective in dissolving tophi that there is even one report of telescoping digits of the hands following the use of allopurinol which resulted in the rapid dissolution of the tophi.[19]

Dietary restrictions for the treatment of gout have long been aban- doned. The French used to forbid German beer. The Germans forbade English ale, and the English forbade French wine. All three agreed that the gouty patient was a high liver and deserved to be punished with severe diet.

SUMMARY

Do not treat hyperuricemia during acute attacks.

TREATMENT OF ACUTE ATTACK

1. Colchicine: oral 0.6 gm tablet two at once, one every hour until diarrhea occurs or IV as one dose of 3 mg, or

2. Phenylbutazone: 200 mg q.i.d. first day, then 100 mg q.i.d., or

3. Indomethacin: 50 mg q.i.d. first day, 25 mg q.i.d. thereafter

INTERVAL TREATMENT: symptomatic colchicine 0.6 mg b.i.d. until symptom free - one year

URICOSURIC AGENTS

1. First Choice: probenecid 0.5 gm - one tablet q.i.d. up to 36 gm daily

2. Second Choice: sulfinpyrazone 100 mg b.i.d. or q.i.d.

3. Third Choice: allopurinol 100-300 mg daily - by far the best but also the most toxic

ASYMPTOMATIC HYPERURICEMIA: TO TREAT OR NOT TO TREAT

"If treated, 'The physician will feel better, if not the patient.'"

T.J. Scott

Hyperuricemia is the hallmark of gout. Although eventually elevated in almost all patients with gout, it may be normal at times. With increasing use of chemical screening as part of the routine physical examination, hyperuricemia is being noted more frequently in asymptomatic patients. There is no general agreement as to whether or not this asymptomatic hyperuricemia should be treated.

It is difficult to differentiate between a normal and an abnormal serum uric acid level. The technique for determining serum uric acid is subject to considerable error. Many common substances spuriously raise the uric level - coffee, vitamin C, acetaminophen and many drugs, particularly diuretics and aspirin in low dosage. Also, the serum uric acid level may vary with age, sex, race, body weight, and from day to day in the same patient. In man, increased uric acid is due to either increased production or decreased excretion. The increased production can be the result of an increase in purine biosynthesis by the body, of an increased catabolism of nucleic acid, or of excessive ingestion of purines. The decreased excretion of uric acid in man is almost always due to a decreased renal clearance.[21] Besides being associated with gout and various drugs, hyperuricemia may also be associated with a number of conditions such as myeloproliferative diseases, chronic hemolytic anemia, renal disfunction, and congestive heart failure.[22]

Untreated hyperuricemia may cause no difficulty in the lifetime of the patient or it may lead to recurrence of acute gouty arthritis, renal stones, and renal failure. On the other hand, the use of uricosuric agents, once started, implies a lifetime of drug therapy that may at times have serious side effects.

To treat or not to treat - no one knows the answer. I am inclined to adhere to the following recommendations of Liang and Fries.[23]

HYPERURICEMIA

1. Normally, an asymptomatic person should not be routinely screened for hyperuricemia. Because the present day standard chemistry screen performed on many patients does screen for hyperuricemia, the problem arises as to whether or not it should be treated or not treated.

2. Before reaching any decision, the finding of hyperuricemia should be confirmed. The standard chemistry screen is a photocolorimetric method which produces false positives. Therefore, the results should be verified by the uricase method, which is accurate.

3. The patient should be carefully questioned and evaluated to determine if the hyperuricemia is secondary to drugs or to blood dyscrasias. If repeated laboratory tests confirm that the patient has significant uric acid elevations and these are not due to secondary factors such as drugs or other diseases, then renal function tests should be done. This should consist

of a serum creatinine and a 24-hour uric acid excretion test. Bear in mind that the 24-hour uric acid excretion test is subject to many variables, such as diet, exercise, and drugs. If the serum creatinine is elevated or if the uric acid excretion exceeds one gram in 24 hours, then there is reason to consider the possibility of treating the hyperuricemia. The elevated creatinine suggests renal damage. The excessive excretion of uric acid suggests the possibility of the risk of development of renal stones. The problem is that no one has demonstrated that hyperuricemia in itself is particularly harmful, while it is well known that drug therapy carries some risk and demands a lifetime of treatment. In this situation, the patient and the physician, after discussing the matter, should reach a decision together. If the decision is made to treat the hyperuricemia, the drug of choice would be allopurinol because this would be the one least likely to cause uric acid stones in the presence of excessive uric acid excretion.

4. If there is significant elevation of uric acid level but no evidence of renal disease and no history of acute arthritis, the patient should be informed of the possible risk of developing an acute arthritis or a renal stone. It would be my recommendation, however, that therapy should be withheld at least until the patient has one acute attack of gouty arthritis.

5. Patients with lymphoproliferation and myeloproliferative disease who have an accompanying hyperuricemia should be treated for this hyperuricemia.

6. Patients with hypertension who have hyperuricemia secondary to thiazide diuretics are not necessarily treated for their hyperuricemia.

The sum total of all of this is that at this point no one is certain as to whether or not the long-term effects of asymptomatic hyperuricemia, when that hyperuricemia is not related to a lymphoma or myeloproliferative disease, should be treated. In favor of the treatment is the possibility that these patients may develop renal stones or gouty arthritis. Against the treatment is the fact that many of these patients never develop any side effects from the hyperuricemia, and once treatment is started, it entails a lifetime of therapy with potential side effects from the drugs. The final decision, therefore, must be made by patient and physician together after discussing the problem.

These guidelines need to be individualized for each patient. Some patients will choose not to decide; others will choose to minimize any risk. In areas of clinical uncertainty such as this, both the physician and patient should be involved in the decision-making process.

REFERENCES

1. Talbot, J.H.: Gout, 2nd Ed., Grune and Stratton, Inc., New York, 1964, p. 117.

2. Holmes, E.W.: Pathogenesis of hyperuricemia in primary gout. In: Clinics in Rheumatic Diseases. W.B. Saunders Co., Philadelphia, 1977.

3. Cannon, P.J., et al.: Hyperuricemia in primary and renal hypertension. The New England Journal of Medicine 275:457, 1966.

4. Steele, T.: Diuretic-induced hyperuricemia. In: Clinics in Rheumatic Diseases. W.B. Saunders Co., Philadelphia, 1977.

5. Goldthwait, J.C., et al.: The diagnoses of gout: Significance of an elevated serum uric acid value. The New England Journal of Medicine 259:1095, 1958.

6. Tabatabi, R.M., et al.: Intravenous colchicine in the treatment of acute pseudogout. Arthritis and Rheumatism 21: 596, 1978.

7. McCarty, D.J., et al.: The significance of calcium phosphate crystals in the synovial fluid of the arthritic patient: The pseudogout syndrome. I. Clinical aspects. Annals of Internal Medicine 56:711, 1962.

8. Schweitz, M.C., et al.: Ibuprofen in the treatment of gouty arthritis. Journal of the American Medical Association 239:34, 1978.

9. Wilkens, R.F., et al.: Treatment of acute gout with naproxen. Journal of Clinical Pharmacology 16:363, 1976.

10. Wallace, S.L.: Colchicine and new anti-inflammatory drugs for the treatment of acute gout. Arthritis and Rheumatism 18:847, 1975.

11. Kaplan, H.: Sarcoid arthritis with a response to colchicine. The New England Journal of Medicine 263:778, 1960.

12. Talbot, J.H. and Coombs, F.S.: Metabolic studies on patients with gout. Journal of the American Medical Association 60:1977, 1938.

13. Yu, T.F. and Gutman, A.B.. Efficacy of colchicine prophylaxis in gout. Annals of Internal Medicine 55:179, 1961.

14. Gutman, A.B. and Yu, T.F.: Benemid as a uricosuric agent in chronic gouty arthritis. Transactions of the Association of American Physicians 64:279, 1951.

15. Talbot, J.H., et al.: The clinical and metabolic effects of Benemid in patients with gout. Transactions of the Association of American Physicians 64:372, 1951.

16. Burns, J.J., et al.: A potent new uricosuric agent, the sulfoxide metabolite of the phenylbutazone analogue, G25671. Journal of Pharmacology and Experimental Therapeutics 119:418, 1957.

17. Yu, T.: Milestones in the treatment of gout. American Journal of Medicine 56:676, 1974.

18. Chawla, S.K., et al.: Allopurinol hepatotoxicity. Arthritis and Rheumatism 20:1546, 1977.

19. Swank, L.E., et al.: Allopurinol-induced granulomatous hepatitis with cholangitis and a sarcoid-like reaction. Archives of Internal Medicine 138:997, 1978.

20. Gottlieb, N.L. and Gray, R.G.: Allopurinol-associated hand and foot deformities in chronic tophaceous gout. Journal of the American Medical Association 238:1663, 1977.

21. Gutman, A.B. and Yu, T.F.: Protracted uricosuric therapy in tophaceous gout. Lancet 2:1258, 1957.

22. Klineberg, J.R.: The management of asymptomatic hyperuricemia. In: Clinics in Rheumatic Diseases. W.B. Saunders Co., Philadelphia, 1977.

23. Liang, M.H. and Fries, J.F.: Asymptomatic hyperuricemia: The case for conservative management. Annals of Internal Medicine 88:66, 1978.

24. Emmerson, B.T.: Hyperuricemia - to treat or not? Practical therapeutics. Drugs 9:141, 1975.

CHAPTER 2: PSEUDOGOUT

CALCIUM PYROPHOSPHATE DIHYDRATE CRYSTAL DEPOSITION DISEASE (CPPD)

McCarty, while working with Hollander studying microcrystals in gouty joint fluid, noted that some of these patients did not have the classic needle-shaped uric acid crystals which he expected to find. Instead, he found rhomboid-shaped crystals which he subsequently identified as calcium pyrophosphate dihydrate crystals, thus discovering and describing a new disease. Because the disease simulated gout, it was called pseudogout.

Subsequent observations carried out by McCarty and his associates and confirmed by other investigators have led to a better understanding of this syndrome. McCarty has suggested that pseudogout should more accurately be called calcium pyrosphosphate dihydrate crystal deposition disease, "CPPD," rather than monosodium urate monohydrate crystal deposition disease, because a specific chemical cause of these conditions has now been identified.

McCarty's original patients were all thought to have gout. Examination of their joint fluid under the microscope using polarized light demonstrated that instead of uric acid crystals, entirely distinct crystals, subsequently identified as calcium pyrophosphate, were present; hence the term pseudogout.

Subsequent studies have demonstrated that there are at least three different types of CPPD crystals. These crystal deposits may occur in about five percent of the adult population and may be related to age. Not all of these people have symptomatic arthritis. It has been recognized that these crystal deposits may be hereditary, sporadic (idiopathic), or associated with metabolic diseases such as hyperparathyroidism, hypothyroidism, diabetes mellitis, and aging.

McCarty now recognizes five different patterns of arthritis associated with CPPD crystal deposits in the cartilage:

TYPE A: PSEUDOGOUT

These patients have acute or subacute attacks of arthritis that resemble the acute attacks of pain associated with the classic uric acid deposition gout. However, the target joint in pseudogout is more likely to be the knee, rather than the toe.

Twenty percent of these patients may have an associated hyperuricemia. Colchicine may provide dramatic relief. Diagnosis, therefore, depends on joint fluid aspiration and examination of the fluid under polarized light microscope for crystals. The pathologist is able to recognize the CPPD crystals as distinct from the uric acid crystals. The radiograph may be of help in demonstrating calcium deposits in the cartilage of the involved joints.

TYPE B: PSEUDORHEUMATOID ARTHRITIS

These patients have multiple joint involvement with subacute attacks and may mimic rheumatoid arthritis in many ways. They complain of morning stiffness, fatigue, and on physical examination there is some synovial thickening, localized edema, limited joint motion, and, in some cases, a positive rheumatoid factor.

TYPES C AND D: PSEUDO-OSTEOARTHRITIS

This group accounts for almost half of McCarty's patients. In these patients, the knees are the most frequently affected joints followed by the wrists, the MCP joints, hips, shoulders, elbows, and ankles. The involvement is usually bilateral and symmetrical. This form of arthritis is distinguished from the usual form of primary osteoarthritis in that CPPD-type disease may in some patients start with exacerbations and remissions. In CPPD disease, there is involvement of the wrists, MCP, elbow, and shoulder joints as contrasted to the typical osteoarthritis, where the involvement is in the terminal phalangeal joints and the first carpometacarpal. The knee is commonly involved in both osteoarthritis and CPPD pseudo-osteoarthritis.

TYPE E: LANTHANIC (Asymptomatic CPPD Crystal Deposition Disease)

This may be the most common type of disease. It may well be that many patients have crystal deposits and are asymptomatic.

TYPE F: PSEUDONEUROTROPHIC JOINTS

A few cases have been described that have a Charcot-like arthropathy of the knee in the absence of neurological abnormality.

Chondrocalcinosis signifies the presence of calcium salt and cartilagenous tissue. Abnormal deposits of these calcium salts can at times be demonstrated radiologically, particularly in the hands of a skilled radiologist.

The diagnosis of CPPD deposition disease is made by a clinical history of acute or chronic synovitis and by the demonstration of CPPD crystals either in joint fluid aspirates or in a joint biopsy. The demonstration of calcification in the cartilage by radiographs is further confirmatory evidence. However, calcification in the cartilage without clinical symptoms cannot be considered diagnostic, because it is unknown how many of these patients are asymptomatic.

The treatment of pseudogout is either by simple joint fluid aspiration or, on occasion, by intra-articular injections of insoluble forms of steroids. Some of these patients will respond to colchicine, much as the patient with gouty arthritis. Most will respond to the various anti-inflammatory agents, particularly indomethacin and phenylbutazone.

SUMMARY

Since the description of pseudogout by McCarty and subsequent workers, it is essential that every patient presenting the diagnosis of acute gouty arthritis have joint fluid aspiration and examination of the joint fluid for specific crystals. It is now apparent that CPPD crystals may be deposited in multiple joints and may be symptomatic, mimicking almost every known form of arthritis. Diagnosis depends on a high degree of suspicion, the demonstration radiologically of calcium deposits in cartilage, and the presence of crystals detected by joint fluid aspiration.

REFERENCES

1. McCarty, D.J. and Hollander, J.L.: Identification of urate crystals in gouty synovial fluid. Annals of Internal Medicine 54:452, 1961.

2. McCarty, D.J., et al.: The significance of calcium pyrophosphate crystals in the synovial fluid of arthritis patients: The pseudogout syndrome. I. Clinical Aspects. Annals of Internal Medicine 56:711, 1962.

3. McCarty, D.J.: Pseudogout: Articular Chondrocalcinosis. Calcium Pyrophosphate Crystal Deposition Disease. In: Arthritis and Allied Conditions, Hollander, J.L., et al. (eds.), Lea and Febiger, Philadelphia, 1972, p. 1140.

4. Suggested Reading: Conference on pseudogout and pyrophosphate metabolism. Arthritis and Rheumatism (Supplement 3) 19:275-507, 1976.

CHAPTER 3: OSTEOARTHRITIS

"If all the patients who claimed back injury
were given $5,000 and advised to spend it
for doctors, lawyers, and drugs, and to keep
the rest for themselves, they would be richer
and the insurance industry would save money."

Anonymous

Degenerative joint disease is the most common disease of all
skeletal animals. It has a wide generic distribution, being found
in those that walk, crawl, swim, or fly. Examples have been
found in dinosaurs, crocodiles, monkeys, birds, ancient species
of horses, and Neanderthal man. The ancient Egyptians were
much afflicted with the disease. Half the adult population over
25 had degenerative disease of the thoracic spine,[1] and recently,
a 3,500-year-old Egyptian mummy was proven to have ochronosis, a form of degenerative arthritis.[2]

It has been estimated that in England, over 80 percent of people
past the age of 55 have radiologic evidence of osteoarthritis[3]
and that a similar incidence exists in the United States.[4] However, this common cause of disability in western civilization receives a minimal amount of attention in textbooks and literature
because it is difficult to study. First of all, there are no known
systemic symptoms or alteration in body chemistries. Secondly,
since the pathology is limited to cartilage and bone, it is almost
impossible to study sequentially in a patient's lifetime. Studies,
therefore, must be primarily limited to autopsies and animal
models. To complicate the matter further, there is no clinical
correlation between radiologic features and symptoms. The most
symptomatic patient may often have normal x-rays, while the
asymptomatic patient shows advanced x-ray changes of osteoarthritis.[5,6]

This most ancient and common disease was not recognized as a
separate entity until 1902. Case records of the Massachusetts
General Hospital prior to 1902 used all-inclusive diagnoses of
rheumatism, acute; rheumatism, chronic; gonorrheal arthritis;

rheumatic gout; and Charcot's joint. Vickery in 1904 recognized it as a separate entity.[7] We still today have not decided on a proper name for the disease. Originally, it was called hypertrophic arthritis, indicating that it was a disease in which there was an overgrowth of bone, distinguishing it from rheumatoid arthritis, then called atrophic arthritis, implying atrophy of the bone. In later years, the term degenerative arthritis was substituted for hypertrophic arthritis. Currently, many people prefer the term osteoarthritis to avoid the implication of a degenerative disease. The English, however, are not willing to accept our nomenclature and insist on osteoarthrosis.[8]

Osteoarthritis is a broad term that encompasses a group of arthritides characterized by cartilage degeneration and bony overgrowth with a relative paucity of inflammatory response in relation to that seen in the other forms of arthritis.[9] For 75 years physicians have been teaching that the disease is a normal process of aging, an inevitable wear-and-tear affair. This has been a facile explanation for both students and patients, but has done little to further research or to clarify the problem and has been grossly unfair to those involved in the medical-legal aspects of the disease.

At the present time, two distinct classifications of this disease are recognized. The bulk of the cases are classified as primary, with no specific etiology apparent. The others are labeled secondary, with an obvious etiology such as trauma, infection, joint abnormality, or other forms of arthritis.

Two pathologic processes occur. First, there is a mechanical disruption of the bearing surface of the articular cartilage, which may be minute at onset and subsequently there is proliferation of the new bone beneath the deteriorating cartilage and at the margins of the bone shafts. Progressive abrasion of the cartilage exposes the underlying bone which becomes polished, and new bone, called osteophyte, forms at the sides of the shafts. Pseudocysts may form directly underneath the polished bone.[10] The pathology of osteoarthritis should be considered as two separate major components: the erosion and destruction of cartilage and the hardening and overgrowth of bone. Although osteoarthritis is considered to be primarily a degenerative disease, synovitis may occasionally occur as a secondary pathologic finding. Synovitis is thought to be caused by the phagocytosis of extruded cartilage particles by the synovial cells with the resulting release of enzymes that stimulate inflammation.[9,11]

Chemically, the articular cartilage is thought today to consist predominantly of collagen and proteoglycans. The proteoglycan is an aggregate consisting of a protein core, which has a polysaccharide-rich portion that contains chondroitin sulfate and keratin sulfate and a polysaccharide-poor portion that interacts with hyaluronic acid. Thirty to forty proteoglycans are linked to each molecule of hyaluronic acid.[12] These protein aggregates are large and a major determinant of the biomechanical properties and physical integrity of the cartilage. Recent studies suggest that, as the result of aging, these compounds lose their ability to form large aggregates, which results in impaired efficiency in aging cartilage.[13]

Ten years ago, Bollet advanced a theory on the etiology of osteoarthritis[14] that is still generally accepted today.[9] Bollet pointed out that there are limited ways in which a tissue can respond to injury and that cartilage degeneration can be produced experimentally by excessive physical stress causing damage to the cartilage. He also noted that cartilage degeneration can be produced by the opposite technique of total immobilization of a joint, thus depriving cartilage of the nutritional influence of intermittent compression. Cartilage is a unique tissue in that there are very few cells floating in a matrix. As there is no blood or nerve supply, the cartilage obtains its nutrition from synovial fluid. Therefore, the metabolic exchange depends on normal use of a joint. The matrix functions like a sponge: as the cartilage is compressed and decompressed, fluid flows out and in.[5] Bollet pointed out that articular cartilage has no nerves. Therefore, the pain associated with osteoarthritis cannot be the direct result of cartilage degeneration. There are pain fibers, however, in the capsule, the ligaments, and the synovial membrane; and it is probable that the secondary alterations which occur in these tissues, plus muscle spasm, contribute to the pain. Since this reaction is inflammatory, it probably accounts for the effectiveness of anti-inflammatory agents in certain cases of osteoarthritis.

Clinically, it is very important to recognize that the symptoms of osteoarthritis show little relationship to the radiologic findings. Although the osteophytes may appear sharp and ominous on x-rays, they are not painful. In the fingers, where the developmental process of Heberden's nodes can be observed before x-ray films reveal spur formation, there is local, pain-producing inflammation at the joint margins. Although fully developed Heberden's nodes may be unattractive cosmetically and radiologically, they seldom hurt. The same process probably occurs in the spine and other joints as well.[14,16] Bollet points out that the following factors should be considered in the etiology of osteoarthritis:

1. Aging of the cartilage is important but is obviously not the entire cause of the disease, since although nearly all of the elderly are afflicted in one joint or another with osteoarthritis, not all their joints are involved simultaneously; nor are the same joints involved in all people, indicating that other contributing factors must exist.

2. Physical stress in cartilage is of importance, but actual weight-bearing is a minor part of this stress, as demonstrated by the rarity of spontaneous osteoarthritis in the ankle joint. Apparently, muscle pull is more stressful and, hence, more destructive than weight-bearing. Once articular disease is present, secondary muscle spasm can increase joint damage.

3. Malalignment - Heavy use of a well aligned joint apparently rarely induces cartilage breakdown. Unusual stresses such as occur with alterations in congruity of articulating surfaces seem to be of most importance. Abnormal stresses occur in joints that are malaligned both congenitally or traumatically, and may account for many of the cases of osteoarthritis. The most common forms of osteoarthritis are chondromalacia of the patella and Heberden's nodes. Neither of these forms of arthritis occurs in weight-bearing joints. The explanation usually offered is that the extensor tendon inserting at the extreme proximal end of the bone, both in the distal phalanx and the patella, produces overextension of the flexed joint causing a considerable mechanical disadvantage and may hasten the development of degenerative changes. One should recognize, however, that not all of Heberden's nodes are the result of the same pathologic process.

4. Genetic factors clearly influence the incidence of osteoarthritis in humans; the disease can be genetically induced in mice. It is important to recognize that posture and joint alignment are, to a large extent, inherited and that structural forces produce physical stresses which precipitate degenerative changes.

5. Systemic diseases, such as diabetes, alkaptonuria, malnutrition, and endocrinopathies (pituitary hormones, estrogen, androgen) influence cartilage metabolism.

The logical conclusion to be drawn from Bollet's theory is that osteoarthritis is a disease of multiple and diverse etiologies with many subgroups.

Osteoarthritis manifests itself clinically by pain. There are no laboratory tests that identify the disease. The symptoms do not parallel x-ray findings. The diagnosis, to a large extent, is based upon the history and physical examination. Objective evidence is present in only a few cases where there is joint swelling and where joint fluid is obtained and found to contain between 1,000 and 2,000 white blood cells. In most cases, the patient describes pain in a few specific joints or in a specific area of the back. It is rare that the pain, which usually is associated with use, is generalized or fleeting. Some jelling and some morning stiffness may be present but are of short duration, five to 15 minutes at the most, as compared to the morning stiffness in inflammatory arthritis which may endure for hours. In the typical case, the patient may have some night pain or morning stiffness but with use is relatively pain-free until, as the joint is used throughout the day, the pain becomes severe. Symptoms of osteoarthritis are also determined by the specific area of the body involved.

THE SPINE

In considering osteoarthritis of the spine, one must be aware that the spine represents multiple complex joints. First, there is the disc cartilage separating each vertebra, held in place by anterior and posterior ligaments, and then there is direct articulation between the vertebrae themselves at the apophyseal joints where the vertebrae join each other. These are synovial joints with fibrous capsules. In the neck there is rotation of the atlas on the axis and in the thoracic region there is union between the transverse processes and the ribs, the costotransverse joints. Degenerative changes which are confined only to the intervertebral discs are referred to as spondylosis and the changes confined to the apophyseal joints are described as degenerative. However, although they both may not be involved in the same vertebra, the two changes usually coexist and the symptoms are inseparable.[17]

LOW LUMBER BACK PAIN

Low lumbar back pain is probably the commonest human complaint and few people will go through life without having some symptoms of low back pain. The condition may be mild and the patient never seek medical attention or it can be severely disabling. The exact cause often defies diagnosis. Low back pain is the major cause of loss of time from work.[18,19] Osteoarthritis of the lumbar spine usually manifests itself by chronic low back pain, a generalized aching, usually without any nerve irritation. Occasionally the pain may be referred to the buttocks, rarely to the hips. It is often associated with night pain. The morning stiffness is of short duration. There is relief with activity and the pain becomes worse as the day wears on. Since radiological abnormalities of osteoarthritis of at least a mild degree occur in almost all individuals 65 or older[20] and since there are no laboratory changes, the diagnosis is based largely on exclusion. The patient with chronic low back pain merits a complete diagnostic workup including standard x-ray examinations of the back, blood count, urinalysis, and chemistry screens because systemic disease may cause chronic low back pain.

In the differential diagnosis, the following conditions are commonly considered:

1. Prolapsed intervertebral disc - Prolapse of a disc usually relates to some stress. It may follow bending, twisting, or lifting and the pain may be so severe that the patient is unable to straighten up. In a few cases the symptoms may develop insidiously after the incident and in some cases there are no precipitating factors. The pain is felt in the back and is referred to the limbs; the distribution and character of the pain vary widely. It can be extremely acute with associated spasm of the back muscles or there may be very little back pain with the major component being the referred pain. Coughing, sneezing, and bowel movements will aggravate the pain and cause a "shooting" of the pain down along the course of the involved nerve root. Spine motion aggravates the pain. The diagnosis depends on finding specific evidence of nerve root involvement, electromyographic studies, and myelogram when indicated.

2. Spondylolisthesis - When there is a defect in both sides of the pars interarticularis of a vertebra and one vertebra slips forward on the other, the condition is known as spondylolisthesis. Originally thought to be congenital, there have been suggestions that it may be the result of repeated injury and trauma.[21] Symptoms of this condition are back pain and stiffness aggravated by motion. Occasionally it is possible to palpate the displaced vertebra on flexion and extension but it is usually diagnosed by the radiograph.

3. Fractures of the various parts of the vertebra do occur and are easily missed. It is important, therefore, in persistent pain, to repeat films in a week or two, particularly where there has been a history of severe trauma.

4. Spinal stenosis - There is considerable variation in the size and shape of the spinal canal. Too narrow a spinal canal

may on rare occasions be a cause of back pain and it is very satisfying to the physician and patient when such a diagnosis can be made. The symptoms are those of peripheral intermittent claudication but the impaired blood supply is to the cauda equina. The patient therefore complains of pain, burning, numbness, and tingling with exercise which are relieved quite readily by rest. If the physician can demonstrate involvement of the cauda equina nerve supply right after exercise, there is good clinical reason to suspect this as the diagnosis. The final diagnosis depends on myelography but is usually not made until surgery when the laminectomy is being performed.

5. The inflammatory arthritides - Rheumatoid spondylitis, Reiter's disease, and sacroileitis secondary to the enteritises may all produce low back pain. They are usually distinguished in that they involve a younger age group. They are associated with prolonged morning stiffness, the positive HLAB-27 antigen, and sclerosis of the sacroiliac joints in the radiograph.

6. Peripheral inflammatory arthritides (rheumatoid and disseminated lupus) are common causes of low back pain, and the diagnosis may be particularly difficult when there is a minimal evidence of peripheral involvement. One should be alerted by the age group, the story of prolonged morning stiffness, laboratory evidence of anemia, an elevated sedimentation rate, and positive serologic tests.

7. Neoplasm and metastatic malignancies are easily missed since they too occur commonly in the older age group. One should be alerted by a physical finding of extreme local tenderness over the vertebrae or the sacroiliac joints. When bone is involved by a metastatic process, simple palpation of the area may cause the patient to scream or jump off the table with pain. An elevated sedimentation rate and anemia in an older person should alert one to trouble, particularly if the chemistry screen shows an elevated alkaline phosphatase. Radioisotope bone scans are helpful in these situations but should be read with caution because trauma may produce an area of increased radioactivity which can easily be mistaken for a metastatic lesion.

8. Paget's disease is probably commoner than is recognized. An elevated alkaline phosphatase should alert the physician to the possibility. The classic x-ray changes of bone destruction and rebuilding are diagnostic.

9. There are a number of metabolic diseases that produce low back pain - hyperparathyroidism, osteoporosis, ochronosis and gout. Although gout is an exceedingly rare cause of low back pain, a few cases have been reported in the literature, and in the presence of hyperuricemia, it is a diagnosis that should be considered. The proof would consist of needling the involved area or biopsying it and obtaining uric acid crystals. Hyperparathyroidism can be recognized by abnormalities of calcium and phosphorus in the chemistry screen, but keep in view the fact that many of these older patients are hypertensive and diuretics may alter the calcium and phosphorus reports. Ochronosis is an exceedingly rare disease characterized by the inability of the body to metabolize normally the aminoacid, tyrosine. There is a congenital absence of homogentisic acid oxidase. Because of the lack of this hormone, homogentisic acid is excreted in the urine. This imparts a brownish black color to the urine when it is alkaline and the patient, usually a male, reports a history of having passed black or smoky urine at times throughout his life. The homogentisic acid can be deposited in the cartilaginous discs between the vertebrae producing a metabolic form of osteoarthritis. The diagnosis depends on the demonstration of homogentisic acid in the urine, and classic x-ray changes described as a wafer calcification and ossification of the intervertebral discs of the lumbar spine. Osteoporosis is a common cause of back pain in the postmenopausal female; and since it can be diagnosed only by x-ray changes and since these changes of bone thinning occur late in the disease, it is probable that many cases of osteoporosis are missed as the cause of back pain.

10. Systemic disease can be a cause of back pain. Any acute infectious process may cause back pain. Gallbladder disease, although it is usually higher than the lumbar spine, may be a factor. Chronic kidney disease should always be considered, although the pain that is described usually suggests a deep organ and is not typical; in view of the fact that some analgesics may cause necrotizing papilitis of the kidneys, the patient who complains of lancinating intermittent low back pain should be suspected of kidney disease. Blood in the urine should alert one to the possibility of chronic kidney disease. Pancreatic disease and deep penetrating peptic ulcers that are chronic may also produce persistent back pain.

11. Sprain - The problem of lumbar sprain is a difficult one. When it occurs following even a minor incident such as lifting

or turning, it may be so devastating that the patient can hardly move. It becomes a problem in industry and in medical legal cases when it persists long after the injury without any specific objective signs of disease. The diagnosis then depends completely on the psychologic evaluation of the patient and his motivation.

The treatment of osteoarthritis of the spine may require hospitalization with traction, physiotherapy, and analgesics in the severe case, although most cases are treated on an ambulatory basis. A hard bed is desirable and this can be easily achieved by placing a quarter-inch thick piece of plywood board between the mattress and the spring. Considerable comfort can be obtained by wearing a lumbosacral belt through the acute phase and after recovery whenever engaging in an activity such as stooping, bending, or lifting that might precipitate or provoke an acute attack. Specific drug therapy varies from adequate doses of aspirin to indomethacin or phenylbutazone (see chapters on these drugs). If the patient does not respond to indomethacin and phenylbutazone, then the diagnosis must be reviewed. These drugs are less likely to be effective if there is nerve involvement. The analgesic drugs may need to be continued for one or two years at minimum maintenance doses. Like other forms of arthritis, the disease has its exacerbations and remissions but symptoms do not go on forever.

Cervical osteoarthritis is as common as osteoarthritis of the lumbar spine. Here, too, radiographic changes and symptoms are not necessarily parallel. At times the radiograph may appear particularly ominous with marked involvement of the foramina, and yet there may be very little evidence of any nerve root involvement. Because of the narrowness of the spinal canal in the cervical spine and because of the multiple branches of nerve roots radiating through the spinal canal, a new dimension is introduced in cervical osteoarthritis, in that cord compression can occur in rare instances and nerve root involvement is frequent.[22]

The symptoms of cervical osteoarthritis are pain, stiffness, night pain, headaches, temporomandibular pain, and limitation of neck motion resulting in driving difficulty. Nerve root involvement may be accompanied by associated radiculopathy. Rarely, an osteophyte protrusion and involvement of the vertebral artery, leading to intermittent dizzy spells particularly associated with head motion, may also be present.

A protruded cervical disc may accompany osteoarthritis, but, particularly in young people, this condition occurs only with trauma, most commonly the so-called "whiplash" injury.[17]

The diagnosis of cervical osteoarthritis demands a complete and thorough examination, because systemic diseases such as osteoporosis, metastatic malignancy, and lesions in the chest, particularly apical tumors and pleural lesions, can manifest themselves as cervical pain. Ordinarily, x-rays of the cervical spine in the AP and oblique positions suffice. A cervical myelogram, never done routinely, is indicated only when there is reasonable suspicion of a possible disc and surgery is contemplated.

In spite of the severity of symptoms, unless there are progressive neurologic symptoms, the disease is treated conservatively. In the most severe cases, hospitalization with traction, heat, analgesics, and sedatives may be indicated. One should not be discouraged by slow progress. Little progress can be seen on a daily basis, and the patient should be advised that he may be in the hospital for one to three weeks. Relief seems to come rather abruptly. Considerable encouragement by the physician is required. Frequently, because of the chronicity of pain and the slowness of relief, the treatment of depression becomes a factor.

The ambulatory patient can be treated with cervical collars. These vary from firm to soft collars and can be fitted by surgical supply stores. The patient should initially be encouraged to wear the collar continuously; as improvement occurs, the collar should be worn only at night. It is well to begin cervical traction under the direction of a physiotherapist who can observe the patient for any possible exacerbation due to treatment. Once the proper amount of cervical traction is known, the patient can be instructed in home use with one of the easily available home devices.

The drugs of choice vary from aspirin, the new anti-inflammatories, and, in severe cases, indomethacin or phenylbutazone. Where there is nerve root involvement, do not expect too much from the anti-inflammatory agents. Because of the severity and disabling nature of many cases of cervical osteoarthritis, there is a temptation to use the stronger analgesics, such as oxycodone with APC (Percodan). These drugs should be administered with extreme caution, particularly in the outpatient. They do offer relief that is far superior to the usual analgesics and anti-inflammatory agents, but the danger of addiction is great and withdrawal is difficult. Many of these patients with cervical pain, particularly in a whiplash injury case where medical-legal problems may arise, may have chronic pain for months. Addicting drugs must be avoided, except in a controlled hospital environment.

Osteoarthritis of the thoracic spine is not common. When it does occur, it may manifest itself by a nerve root pain. At the onset, one should carefully watch the patient for the development of herpes zoster, particularly if the pain is unilateral. If the pain is at all atypical, one must consider the possibility of gallbladder disease, pancreatic disease, liver disease, renal disease, osteoporosis, or a metastatic malignancy. Most cases of clear-cut osteoarthritis of the thoracic spine will respond to analgesics and anti-inflammatory agents.

Osteoarthritis of the temporomandibular joint is a common affliction. The average patient is usually seen by the dentist or oral surgeon and, as a result, most physicians are under the illusion that the condition hardly exists. The contrary is the case. The condition can be more disabling than almost any other form of degenerative arthritis, because it interferes with eating and talking. Temporomandibular joint involvement manifests itself by pain, difficulty in opening the mouth, and, with progression, ankylosis of the joint, making it almost impossible to open the mouth. Additionally, symptoms may be referred to the ear, causing hearing impairment, tinnitus, dizziness, and stuffy sensations in the ear; occipital headaches may also occur.

Physical examination may reveal mandibular hypomobility and deviation on opening. Muscle tenderness may also be found locally, and a clicking of the jaw is a frequent sign.

Radiologic examination of the temporomandibular joint is difficult and requires special technique by trained personnel with the proper equipment. Radiographs are taken in the closed and open mouth positions, and, in some instances tomograms are indicated.

The temporomandibular joint is a complicated joint anatomically, consisting of two compartments and two motions. The joint movement consists of an opening motion which is pure rotation around a horizontal axis, and when the maximum opening is achieved, further opening depends upon gliding.

Temporomandibular joint disease falls into two large groups: those with organic joint abnormalities which are secondary to trauma or infectious arthritis, and those that are secondary to functional disease. The patient with functional disease, however, with repeated abnormal jaw movements, muscle spasms, and teeth grinding, can develop a secondary degenerative arthritis. Almost all temporomandibular afflictions are accompanied by abnormalities in the bite which may be a primary cause or a secondary development.

The treatment of a temporomandibular joint pain should involve a knowledgeable dentist to correct bite problems. Temporary relief can be obtained with analgesics, physiotherapy, heat, ultrasound, sedatives, and splints to correct the bite. In a few cases, surgery may be necessary.[23]

Involvement of the hands is one of the most common forms of osteoarthritis. When involving the terminal phalangeal joints, it is termed Heberden's node; when involving the proximal interphalangeal joint, it is called Bouchard's nodes. It is usually a familial disease of middle and advancing life, and for some unknown reason occurs more often in women than in men. The symptoms may develop insidiously with little pain or may be marked by an acute inflammatory process with redness, tenderness, swelling and considerable pain. The patient may well complain of paresthesia, clumsiness in the use of the hands or fingers, or difficulty in daily tasks involving fine use of the fingers, such as writing or typing. Soft cartilaginous nodes may develop near the joint. These are gelatinous cysts, often attached to tendon sheaths, which may persist indefinitely or recede spontaneously. As the disease progresses, the pain eventually disappears, but joint destruction, dislocated terminal phalangeal joints, stiffness in the hands, and difficulty in participating in sports requiring hand use may remain. The first carpometacarpal joint (the base of the thumb) is frequently involved.

As the disease progresses the increasing cosmetic deformity may be a major problem.[24]

When the proximal interphalangeal joints are involved, osteoarthritis may resemble rheumatoid arthritis. The distinction is usually not difficult, because in osteoarthritis there are no laboratory changes, no systemic symptoms, and no other joint involvement.

As for treatment, the most important aspect of the therapy is reassurance of the patient. From the initial visit the patient should be informed that he does not have a spreading, crippling form of arthritis. Because of the cosmetic changes, many patients inquire about surgery. No surgical procedure can be satisfactorily recommended. The gelatinous cyst may recur if removed, and such removal may be much more complicated than the removal of a simple cyst. As for drug therapy, it is my custom to advise the patient that since we are dealing with a benign disease, treatment to a large extent can be determined by the patient's pain tolerance threshold. If the patient is comfortable with simple aspirin, then nothing more should be done. In the occasional severe case where the patient's occupation requires hand use, the nonsteroidal anti-inflammatory agents, indomethacin or phenylbutazone might be indicated. Physical therapy in the form of home paraffin baths offers symptomatic relief. During acute phases, a small hypodermic injection of insoluble steroids may give prolonged relief. Many of my patients have found symptomatic relief during acute phases with nightly splinting. This can be accomplished by the use of a tongue blade or a dessert stick and adhesive tape. One of my ingenious patients sewed pockets in the fingers of white flannel gloves and slipped the dessert sticks into the pockets and wore the gloves at night.

The first metatarsophalangeal joint of the foot is frequently involved in osteoarthritis. Usually the symptom is slowly progressive; the diagnosis is established by noting the painful swollen joint, the distortion of the joint, and x-ray changes. The symptom can usually be relieved by properly fitting shoes.

When osteoarthritis occurs in the weight-bearing joints, the knee or the hip, it can be disabling to the point of crippling. Osteoarthritis of the hip manifests itself primarily by pain with use. The pain may be referred to the groin and on occasion into the knee. Stiffness and night pain may exist but do not approach the severity and duration of the pain characteristic of rheumatoid involvement of the hip. The diagnosis rests on the patient's history of pain and radiographic evidence of degeneration of the cartilage and osteophyte formation. At the onset of the disease, x-rays may be negative. Because of the severity and the disabling nature of osteoarthritis of the hip, therapy should be aggressive. The patient should be told that increased pain and disability will follow increased hip use. The patient may have difficulty accepting this concept, which seems to contradict the patient's experience. The physician should explain, however, that the pain that follows the use of the joint indicates further joint damage. In severe cases of osteoarthritis in the hip, bed rest for a period of a few weeks to lessen the severity of symptoms may be essential.

The use of a cane to remove tremendous amounts of weight bearing from the hip is invaluable. The cane should be carried in the hand opposite the afflicted side.

Osteoarthritis of the hip seldom responds to minor analgesics and anti-inflammatory agents. Indomethacin and phenylbutazone are particularly effective here. The ultimate solution, and one that can be very satisfying, is total hip replacement, but this should be recommended only in advanced cases (see Part Three, Chapter 6, Surgery in Arthritis).

Osteoarthritis of the knee is as disabling as osteoarthritis of the hip. It manifests by pain and occasionally by swelling of the knee. When swelling is present, diagnostic aspiration of the joint fluid for crystal examination is helpful; a low white count helps to confirm the diagnosis of osteoarthritis. The roentgenogram is of value in showing the progression of the disease and indicating whether the disease involves both the medial and lateral compartments of the knee or only one compartment. The treatment of osteoarthritis of the knee involves rest, the use of a cane, and the use of knee supports. The simple elastic support is of no value because the material does not retain its firmness for a sufficient length of time. Instead, one should recommend an elastic knee support with hinged metal sides. These can be obtained inexpensively from mail order catalogs. Better fitting ones can be obtained at orthopedic and surgical supply stores. One version is made with leather which can be laced to fit and correspond exactly to the joint. In general, it is advisable not to wear an elastic knee support for long periods of sitting, such as on airplanes or in cars, because of the possibility of edema of the lower extremity.

Intra-articular injections of insoluble steroids offer such dramatic relief in osteoarthritis of the knee that one is tempted to repeat them endlessly. However, repeated injections are contraindicated and may lead to joint overuse, thus hastening the destruction of the cartilage. In addition, as we approach the era of artificial joint replacement, the danger of infection in the knee joint must be considered. A latent infection could result in disaster if surgery is later contemplated.

As in other forms of osteoarthritis, the analgesic of choice depends on the severity of pain and ranges from aspirin to the newer anti-inflammatory agents, indomethacin and phenylbutazone.

A temporizing surgery in osteoarthritis of the knee when the disease is confined to only one compartment is osteotomy. This should be particularly considered in the younger patient (see Part Three, Chapter 6, Surgery in Arthritis).

Primary osteoarthritis of the shoulder, elbow, wrist and ankle is rare. When these joints are involved, one should consider seeking a causation.

In 1952, Kellgren and Moore described a form of generalized polyarthritis which had some of the characteristics of an inflammatory arthritis but which was actually a form of generalized osteoarthritis. In this disease, there is inflammatory involvement of the small hand joints which resembles the involvement seen in osteoarthritis of the hands; but in addition there is involvement of the large joints - the knees and the hips and often the vertebral column. It differs from the usual form of osteoarthritis in that there is multiple joint involvement. It is distinguished from rheumatoid arthritis by a normal or only slightly elevated sedimentation rate and by negative agglutination tests.[25]

One form of osteoarthritis is known as erosive or inflammatory arthritis. The terms were introduced by Peter and Ehrlich to describe an inflammatory condition of the interphalangeal joints of the hand. In the characteristic case, inflammation of these joints precedes the development of a progressive, deforming osteoarthritis, and subsequent x-ray examinations show both degenerative changes (joint space narrowing and osteophyte formation) and erosions. It is sometimes difficult to distinguish the disease from rheumatoid arthritis, but the absence of positive laboratory tests and the limitation of the pathology to the hands ultimately makes the diagnosis apparent. Treatment is the same as for other forms of osteoarthritis of the hands. Local steroid injections offer temporary relief but do not alter the course of the disease.[26]

Secondary osteoarthritis refers to forms of the disease in which an etiologic factor can be demonstrated. Trauma is usually considered as a cause, but normal joint use does not cause joint destruction. Exercise is essential for normal nutrition of articular cartilage. The point at which exercise and internal stresses to a joint result in harm is unknown, and it is conceivable that in a normal joint this point may never be reached. Direct trauma to a joint can produce arthritis. The classic example of this is the "baseball finger." Overtraining, overuse, and direct injury in sports are known to be associated with osteoarthritis. There are reports describing osteoarthritis in the knees and ankles in football players; the spine in judo participants; the hands in boxers; the shoulders and elbows in baseball pitchers; the patella in cyclists; the spine, knees and elbows in wrestlers; the fingers in cricketeers; the shoulders, elbows, and wrists in gymnasts; and the ankles and knees in lacrosse players.[27]

Occupations, as well as sports, have been associated with osteoarthritis: the elbows and knees in miners, the ankles and feet in ballet dancers, the fingers in cotton pickers, the shoulders and elbows in pneumatic drill operators and the hips in farmers.[28]

There are local causes for osteoarthritis. One of the most troublesome is aseptic necrosis (avascular necrosis) due to an impaired blood supply to the femoral head. The exact cause for the interruption of blood supply is unknown, but the patient complains bitterly of severe hip pain on active and passive motion. Initial radiographic examinations may be normal but, if repeated within a few weeks, show complete dissolution of the femoral head and a wedge formation. The patient is almost totally disabled. Aseptic necrosis has been associated with trauma, usually a fracture or a subluxation, corticosteroid therapy, systemic lupus erythematosus, rheumatoid arthritis, scleroderma, pancreatitis, alcoholism, sickle cell anemia, and Gaucher's disease.[28]

Congenital abnormalities of the hip, with the resulting abnormalities in joint structure and the development of abnormal lines of stress, account for from 20 to 50 percent of the cases of osteoarthritis of the hip. Legg-Perthes disease and slipped femoral epiphyses are common congenital conditions which are forerunners of degenerative joint disease.[29]

Neuropathic diseases which result in severe trauma because of the loss of protective proprioceptive mechanisms can lead to the development of Charcot's joints, a form of degenerative arthritis. The usual diseases that may be involved are tabes dorsalis, diabetes mellitus and syringomyelia.[30]

Inflammatory arthritis is a well recognized cause of osteoarthritis. The initial pathology, for example, may be rheumatoid arthritis; as the disease progresses, the degenerative changes may overshadow the inflammatory changes and may be the cause of major symptoms. Both septic arthritis and tuberculosis may eventually lead to osteoarthritis.

Hemophilia is commonly complicated by osteoarthritis. The joints most frequently involved are the elbows and the knees. The pathology is caused by repeated hemorrhages into the synovium and into subchondral bone with subsequent pannus formation and cartilage destruction. A particularly notable radiologic feature, especially in the tibia, is severe subchondral bone destruction and cyst formation.

Hemochromatosis and Wilson's disease may be complicated by osteoarthritis which is probably caused by abnormal deposits of iron. A similar form of arthritis has been described in secondary hemosiderosis and has been produced experimentally in rabbits following iron administration.

Alkaptonuria (ochronosis) is a metabolic disease associated with an excretion of homogentisic acid in the urine and the binding of this acid to connective tissue components. An abnormal deposit of one of the pigments of this acid in the cartilage might possibly lead to the generalized osteoarthritis involving the spine.[24]

Spondyloepiphyseal dysplasia is a very rare disease in which large quantities of keratin sulfate are excreted in the urine, resulting in gross skeletal deformities. There is epiphyseal dysplasia and fragmentation of the articular cartilage.[30]

A form of osteoarthritis has been recognized in Kashin-Beck disease. This is a disorder in growing children endemic to certain regions of Siberia, Mongolia and North Korea and has been attributed to the ingestion of grain contaminated with a fungus. Its importance lies in demonstrating that there may be nutritional factors or infectious factors in the pathogenesis of osteoarthritis.

Obesity has been found to be associated with an increased instance of osteoarthritis. Surprisingly, it is apparently not caused by excessive weight on the weight-bearing joints, because it can also involve other nonweight-bearing joints, such as those of the hands. This suggests metabolic factors.

An increased incidence of osteoarthritis has also been reported in patients with diabetes mellitus.[30]

Crystal-induced arthropathy can occur (see Part Two, Chapters 1 and 2, Gout and Pseudogout). Uric acid deposits in joints may be followed by degenerative changes. McCarthy, since his description of pseudogout, has now recognized that there are multiple forms of arthritis associated with chondrocalcinosis. In five percent of the patients in his series, multiple joint involvement has occurred with subacute attacks lasting from four weeks to several months. Nonspecific symptoms of inflammation, such as morning stiffness and fatigue, are common. Signs such as synovial thickening, localized pitting edema, limitation of joint motion due to inflammation, flexion contractors, and elevated erythrocyte sedimentation rate are found. These patients are often initially diagnosed as having rheumatoid arthritis, but the rheumatoid factor is very rare in this type of crystal-induced arthritis. The most important diagnostic point is the aspiration of crystals from the joint and the radiologic evidence of calcification in the cartilage.[31]

SUMMARY

Osteoarthritis is a disease characterized by erosion of cartilage, progressive destruction of the cartilage with narrowing of joint space and subsequent hardening of the bone beneath the cartilage, and the development of bony overgrowths called osteophytes. The predominant symptom is pain with use associated with stiffness of short duration. The disease is usually local with few joints involved and localized symptoms which may be compounded by nerve root involvement when the cervical or lumbar spine is involved. Usually, the disease is idiopathic and hence called primary osteoarthritis, but no increasingly recognized secondary form exists in which a specific etiologic agent such as congenital abnormality or metabolic, endocrine, or genetic factors can be demonstrated to be an etiologic cause. Since the disease is not crippling if the major weight-bearing joints are not involved, treatment is usually symptomatic and should be limited to the minor inflammatory agents. In the severe cases, indomethacin or phenylbutazone is used. Surgery may be necessary in a small percentage of cases.

THE EXPERT MEDICAL WITNESS
CONCERNING OSTEOARTHRITIS

"It seems reasonable to assume that if you want to understand how the joint breaks down, you might try to understand how it normally works. Attempts to do this in synovial joints have been sadly lacking, and to my knowledge no physiology textbook or arthritis textbook as yet treats the subject of joint physiology in any detail . . . I am indebted to Rodnan for reviewing the early literature and for finding Bichat's nineteenth century remark, 'No part of the physiology of the bones abounds more in hypotheses and less in discoveries than the history of the synovial system.' This still ranks as an understatement."[32]

Osteoarthritis, because of its frequency and involvement in injury, is one of the most common areas of expert medical testimony. For 75 years the medical expert has generally described it as a "wear-and-tear" disease. Only recently has medical research been initiated in this area. It would appear that it is time to reevaluate the medical position.

For those interested in becoming true experts on the problem of osteoarthritis, I would suggest initially reading the works of Radin,[32,33] the papers by Howell and Moskowitz,[9] the review by Lee and colleagues,[28] Bollet's work,[14] and the editorial by Moskowitz.[34]

The expert should consider the following points:

1. There is general agreement that symptoms and x-ray changes are not necessarily parallel. The older the patient, the more likely are x-ray changes. In the majority of patients, there are no symptoms.

2. Cartilage aging and the x-ray changes of osteoarthritis are a normal occurrence in older patients.

3. Normal physical stresses such as walking and weight-bearing do not produce degenerative changes in a normal joint.

4. Impact loading, that is, sudden repeated stresses, may be a factor in degenerative arthritis in a susceptible joint. Heavy use of a well aligned joint rarely induces cartilage breakdown, but osteoarthritis can be seen in the hind limbs of older draft horses who perform hard labor with their hind limbs and young thoroughbred racehorses whose forelimbs are subject to great concussive forces.

5. Direct trauma to a joint can cause osteoarthritis, as exemplified by the baseball finger. Increased evidence of involvement of specific joints in certain types of sports is probably more often related to trauma than to impact loading.

6. Osteoarthritis of the shoulder, elbow, wrist, and ankle is seldom primary. In such instances, always look for a cause.

7. Osteoarthritis is associated with various joint involvement in specific occupations, the classic example being the shoulder and hand involvement in the pneumatic drill operator.

8. In recent years, much evidence has accumulated to suggest that an inherited predisposition may be an important factor in the causation of human osteoarthritis. Congenital abnormalities which result in abnormal joint alignment may be a common cause of osteoarthritis of the hip, an example of which would be congenital dysplasia of the hip with or without dislocation.

9. Obesity apparently plays a factor in the development of osteoarthritis. It is due not to weight-bearing, but rather to some metabolic changes.

10. Endocrine abnormalities are probably involved. There is evidence that testosterone hastens the development of osteoarthritis and estrogen may delay it.

11. Osteoarthritis has been caused by eating foods contaminated with fungi.

12. Osteoarthritis may be secondary to early inflammatory polyarthritides, examples of which are rheumatoid arthritis, Reiter's disease, spondylitis, and gout.

Subtle x-ray changes that suggest an etiology other than trauma and stress may be present and are as follows:[35]

1. Overgrowth of soft tissues occurs secondary to excessive growth hormone levels in acromegaly and can cause a generalized increase in the thickness of the skin and subcutaneous tissues of the hands.

2. Abnormal calcific deposits suggest metabolic disease or scleroderma.

3. When erosions accompany osteoarthritic changes, one should consider a generalized osteoarthritis, such as Kellgren's or erosive osteoarthritis.

4. Ectopic bone formation associated with degenerative changes suggests an osteoarthritis secondary to neurotropic changes (Charcot's joint).

5. Where the joint disease is suspected to be secondary to trauma, it is worthwhile x-raying the other parallel joint, which was not subjected to trauma. Equally degenerative changes in both joints would suggest factors other than trauma as being the etiologic cause.

6. When degenerative changes in the foot are accompanied by erosions, consider gout.

7. The ankle - Heel spurs are usually associated with Reiter's syndrome or ankylosing spondylitis. Proliferative spurs are usually associated with flat feet (pes cavus).

8. The knee - Calcification of the cartilage of the knee or, for that matter, of any joint should suggest chondrocalcinosis. Calcification in the knee joint space may represent any of four entities: calcification of the synovium, calcification of cartilage, calcification of cruciate ligaments, or the presence of a fragment of bone. There is debate as to whether these conditions are the result of localized trauma or represent areas of localized inflammation with resulting calcification.

9. Abnormalities of alignment in the lower extremity - The axis of the femur and the tibia should be on a 180º line with each other. Any deviation is abnormal and results in a condition known as knocked knees or bowed legs, depending upon the alignment. Abnormal alignment will be a factor in future degenerative development. The most common malalignment seen in the hip is an abnormal angle between the shaft of the femur and its neck. Normally, this angle is between 120º to 130º. Changes in this angle will result in degenerative changes and are usually the result of an underlying congenital defect, osteomalacia, or Paget's disease.

10. The spine - Involvement of multiple disc spaces suggests a metabolic disease such as ochronosis. Involvement of the sacroiliac suggests an inflammatory arthritis.

REFERENCES

1. Wells, C.F.A.: Bones, Bodies and Disease. Prayer Book Press, Bridgeport, Ct., 1964, p. 54.

2. Lee, S.L., et al.: Characterization of mummy bone ochronotic pigment. Journal of the American Medical Association 240:136, 1978.

3. Kellgren, J.H.: Osteoarthritis and disc degeneration in an urban population. Annals of Rheumatic Diseases 16:494, 1957.

4. Gordon, T.: Osteoarthrosis in U.S. Adults. In: Population Studies of the Rheumatic Diseases. Bennet, ·P.H. and Wood, P.H.N., (eds.), Excerpta Medica Foundation, Princeton, N.J., 1968, p. 391.

5. Wood, P.H.N.: Rheumatic complaints. British Medical Bulletin 27:82, 1971.

6. Kellgren, J.H., et al.: Rheumatism in miners, Part II: X-ray study. British Journal of Industrial Medicine 9:197, 1952.

7. Vickery, N.F.: Chronic joint disease at the Massachusetts General Hospital. Boston Medical and Surgical Journal 151: 536, 1904.

8. Goldthwait, J.E.: The differential diagnoses and treatment of the so-called rheumatic diseases. Boston Medical and Surgical Journal 151:529, 1904.

9. Howell, D.S. and Moskowitz, R.W.: Introduction: Symposium on osteoarthritis. Arthritis and Rheumatism 20 (Supplement) : 596, 1977.

10. Sokoloff, L. and Bland, J.N.: The Musculoskeletal System. The Williams and Wilkins Co., Baltimore, 1975, p. 128.

11. Chrisman, O.P.: Experimental production of synovitis and marginal articular exostosis in knee joint of dogs. Yale Journal of Biological Medicine 37:409, 1965.

12. Perricone, E., et al.: Failure of proteoglycans to form aggregates in morphologically normal-aged human hip cartilage. Arthritis and Rheumatism 20:1372, 1977.

13. Greenwald, R.A., et al.: Functional properties of cartilage proteoglycans. Seminars in Arthritis and Rheumatism 8:53, 1978.

14. Bollet, J.A.: An essay on the biology of osteoarthritis. Arthritis and Rheumatism 12:152, 1969.

15. Linn, F.C. and Sokoloff, L.: Movement and composition of interstitial fluid of cartilage. Arthritis and Rheumatism 8: 481, 1965.

16. Lawrence, J.S., et al.: Osteoarthrosis, prevalence in the population and relationship between symptoms and x-ray changes. Annals of Rheumatic Disease 25:1-24, 1966.

17. Jayson, M.I.V.: Degenerative disease of the spine and back. Clinics in Rheumatic Disease 2:557, 1976.

18. Wilson, P.D., Jr.: Low back pain. A problem for industry. Archives of Environmental Health 5:505, 1962.

19. Benn, R.T. and Wood, P.H.N.: Pain in the back: An attempt to estimate the size of the problem.
and Rehabilitation 14:128, 1964.

20. Lawrence, J.S.: Osteoarthritis prevalence in the population and relationship between symptoms and x-ray changes. Annals of Rheumatic Disease 25:1, 1966.

21. Wiltse, L.L., et al.: Fatigue fracture: The basic lesion in isthmic spondylolisthesis. Journal of Bone and Joint Surgery 57A:17, 1975.

22. Lawrence, J.S., et al.: The Epidemiology of Chronic Rheumatism. Kellgren, J.H., et al., (eds.), Vol. I, Blackwell Scientific Publications, Philadelphia, 1963.

23. Guralhick, W., et al.: Temporomandibular joint afflictions. The New England Journal of Medicine 299:123, 1978.

24. Moskowitz, R.W.: Clinical and Laboratory Findings in Osteoarthritis. In: Arthritis, 8th Ed., Hollander, J.L., McCarty, D.J., (eds.), Lea and Febiger, Philadelphia, 1972, p. 1034.

25. Kellgren, J.H. and Moore, R.: Generalized osteoarthritis and Heberden's nodes. British Medical Journal 1:181, 1952.

26. Utsiner, P.D., et al.: Roentgenologic, immunologic and therapeutic study of erosive arthritis (inflammatory osteoarthritis). Archives of Internal Medicine 138:693, 1978.

27. Adams, I.D.: Osteoarthritis and Sports. In: Clinics in Rheumatic Disease. W.B. Saunders Co., Philadelphia, 1976.

28. Lee, P., et al.: The etiology and pathogenesis of osteoarthrosis: A review of seminars. Arthritis and Rheumatism 3:189, 1974.

29. Adam, A., et al.: Intertrochanteric osteotomy for osteoarthrosis of the hip. Journal of Bone and Joint Surgery 40B: 219, 1958.

30. Eloesser, L.: Neuropathic defections of joints. Annals of Surgery 66:201, 1917.

31. McCarty, D.J.: Calcium Pyrophosphate Dihydrate Crystal Deposition Disease. In: Clinics in Rheumatic Disease. W.B. Saunders Co., Philadelphia, 1977.

32. Radin, E.L.: The physiology and degeneration of joints. Seminars in Arthritis and Rheumatism 2:245, 1973.

33. Radin, E.L.: Etiology of osteoarthrosis. Clinics in Rheumatic Disease 2:509, 1973.

34. Moskowitz, R.W.: Cartilage and osteoarthritis: Current concepts. Journal of Rheumatology 4:4, 1977.

35. Forrester, D.M. and Nesson, J.W.: The Radiology of Joint Disease. W.B. Saunders Co., Philadelphia, 1973.

CHAPTER 4: RHEUMATOID ARTHRITIS

"The hand of the patient with rheumatoid arthritis is his calling card."

Phillip Hench

Rheumatoid arthritis is usually thought of as a chronic progressive systemic disease of young women, characterized by peripheral joint involvement, marked morning stiffness, fatigue, anemia, and elevated sedimentation rate.

The disease can involve either sex and any age group, can occasionally start as a monoarticular disease, and can in some cases start with exacerbations and remissions. To complicate the matter even further, it is now recognized that other forms of arthritis, such as osteoarthritis, arthritis associated with chronic bowel disease, spondylitis, infectious arthritis, and even gout, may mimic rheumatoid arthritis.

Seventy percent of the cases occur between the ages of 25 and 54. Three cases out of four occur in the female.

The etiology of the disease is still unknown. Originally, when rheumatoid arthritis was distinguished from the other forms of rheumatism, it was called atrophic arthritis, in contrast to osteoarthritis which was called hypertrophic arthritis. The term atrophic was meant to apply to the muscle and joint atrophy which developed as the disease progressed. The name was subsequently changed to rheumatoid arthritis, implying that it was inflammatory in nature. In the late 1930s and early 1940s, it was often unofficially referred to as C.I.A., chronic infectious arthritis, implying that there was a specific infectious etiology. However, with the development of antibiotic therapy and the failure of the disease to respond to any antibiotic, the term chronic infectious arthritis was dropped.

Clinically, rheumatologists had noted that approximately one third of the patients described stressful life situations occurring prior to the development of their arthritis. They were also aware

that many patients with rheumatoid arthritis subjected to prolonged emotional or physical stress had an exacerbation of their
disease. In the middle 1940s, the work of Selye demonstrating
the effect of stress on animals popularized the theory that stress
was an important factor in the development of rheumatoid arthritis. This theory, however, has long been abandoned, because the disease has never been produced experimentally by
stress.

There is no evidence that climate is a major factor in the disease. The disease occurs in all races and in all environments.

Pregnancy and jaundice both are known to cause remission in the
symptoms of rheumatoid arthritis. This suggests the role of
hormones, but unfortunately excessive use of hormones has not
resulted in altering the course of the disease.

The current theory as to the etiology of the disease is that it
represents "an autoimmune disease," a condition in which the
lymphocytes of the body are out of balance or control, have lost
the ability of "self-recognition," and attack the connective tissue; the organism is on a program of self-destruct. Once more
we have gone full circle, and again the theory that this may be
an infectious arthritis is popular. The suggestion is that either
a virus or a specific bacterium initially triggers the abnormality in a genetically predisposed individual.

At this time all is theory. The disease manifests itself in a variety of ways in different individuals. In some patients the extra-articular manifestations may be more obvious than the joint
manifestations; some patients have rheumatoid factors in their
sera, some patients lack rheumatoid factors, some patients
have a rapidly destructive progressive disease, some have the
disease in an indolent, slowly progressing form. It is this di-
versity of symptoms that raises the question as to whether the
disease has multiple etiologies or one etiology with the variation
being due to the differences in the reacting host. [1-6]

Pathologically, the earliest changes occur in the synovial mem-
branes which show signs of inflammation and infiltration with
lymphocytes and plasma cells. Ultimately there is proliferation
of the synovial cells leading to villae formation and joint effusion.
Inflammation also occurs in the joint capsule, bursa, tendon,
and tendon sheaths. As the disease progresses, the synovial
membrane becomes thickened and fibrotic, and the cartilage is
eroded by the overgrowth of the granulation tissue from the pe-
riphery. Ultimately there is erosion of the underlying bone, lig-
ament destruction, and subluxation of the joints. The major

extra-articular lesion is a subcutaneous nodule. There may be widespread involvement of connective tissue anywhere in the body, leading to pleurisy, pericarditis, arteritis, eye involvement, lung involvement, cardiac and pericardial involvement, neuritis, myositis.

The clinical course is variable. Often fatigue is a prodromal symptom; and because this fatigue is in a young woman in whom there is no physical or laboratory evidence of disease, it is diagnosed as a functional illness.

In most cases the joint involvement is symmetrical from the onset. First the small joints of the hands, the metacarpal phalangeal, and the proximal interphalangeal joints become swollen and tender. This may be accompanied by involvement of the metatarsal joints of the feet. The terminal phalangeal joints of the hands are never involved. Once started, the disease tends to be chronic and progressive with subsequent involvement of other joints. No joint in the body is safe.

In a small percentage of the patients, the onset may be acute with fever, anorexia, weight loss, and marked signs of inflammation in the joints.

An unusual onset may be a monoarticular arthritis such as a shoulder joint or a knee. This type of onset is particularly confusing because it is usually considered to be traumatic or infectious and can only be diagnosed by biopsy or subsequent course; joint fluid aspiration provides an important clue.

A few rare cases start with exacerbations and remissions and remissions and normal laboratory tests, so they are labeled palindromic rheumatism; or, because signs and symptoms may be absent when the patient is examined, they are misdiagnosed as psychogenic rheumatism.

One of the most important diagnostic symptoms is the patient's voluntary description of morning stiffness. In the typical case, the patient describes aching and stiffness throughout the night with marked morning stiffness on arising so that it is difficult to get out of bed. Often the patient can get out of bed only with help. A hot shower helps and activity relieves the morning stiffness. The morning stiffness is usually of long duration, one or two hours or possibly almost all day. An accompanying symptom is labeled "jelling." The patient describes aching and stiffness when sitting for a long period of time such as in a theater or on an automobile ride.

The RA test (Rheumatoid Factor), agglutination of sensitized sheep erythrocytes by the sera of patients with rheumatoid arthritis, was first described by Meyer and later by Waaler. In 1948, Rose and his colleagues devised a diagnostic test for rheumatoid arthritis based on this reaction. It has since undergone a number of modifications.[7] In the original test, the sheep cell was treated with sensitized rabbit serum and then an agglutination test was undertaken with the patient's serum. This actually was a very inexact and cumbersome test and primarily of value in a research laboratory until it was modified by the use of latex particles. The inert latex particles are treated with a gamma globulin mixture and tested with progressive dilutions of serum. The test has become known as the latex fixation test.[8] The test determines the presence of rheumatoid factor which is an antigamma globulin. The common procedure used is a slide test which is obtainable as a kit; it can be performed in most laboratories. An agglutination reaction occurs if the rheumatoid factor is present. The test is done routinely on all patients in whom rheumatoid arthritis is suspected. It should not be used as a prime diagnostic test because it is positive in about 80 percent of the patients with rheumatoid arthritis, but 20 percent of the patients in whom a test is negative still have a rheumatoid arthritis which is indistinguishable from those with a positive test. In addition, a positive test can occur in approximately five percent of the normal population. The positive rheumatoid factor occurs in a number of diseases other than rheumatoid arthritis. It is estimated that over 90 percent of the patients with Sjogren's syndrome have rheumatoid factor; 30 percent of the patients with systemic lupus erythematosus also have a positive factor. A positive factor is frequently found in subacute bacterial endocarditis, tuberculosis, leprosy, scleroderma, polymyositis, chronic hepatitis, pulmonary fibrosis, syphilis, sarcoidosis, and many other chronic diseases.[9,10]

THE RADIOGRAPH

It is the early radiologic signs of rheumatoid arthritis that are the most difficult to detect and the most important diagnostically. The following are some of the early signs to look for.[11]

1. Soft tissue changes: These are usually the first objective radiologic evidence of disease and indicate to the radiologist where one should look for bone changes.

2. Bone rarefaction: Rarefaction of bone occurs due to decreased use caused by pain. It is best detected by comparing

bilateral symmetrical regions. It is therefore wise to order radiographs of the contralateral regions even if they are unaffected.

3. Periosteal ossification: Inflammation involving a bone will involve the contiguous periosteum. The periosteum becomes edematous and eventually calcified. These changes should be looked for especially in the metacarpophalangeal joint or the ankle joint.

4. Erosions: Erosions are the most definitive radiologic changes. The erosions may occur on the joint surface or just beneath the joint surface but they are always near the joint, never in the shaft of the bone.

5. Narrowed joint space: The narrowing of the joint space implies a loss of articular cartilage. It is usually first apparent in the interphalangeal joints and in the wrist, carpus, tarsus, knee, and hip.

A complete physical examination is essential in every patient suspected of having rheumatoid arthritis. Not only does it aid in diagnosis but it determines a baseline to follow the subsequent course of the patient. The extra-articular examination is as essential as the examination of the joints because the finding of nodules, tophi, enlarged spleen, or a cardiac murmur may point the direction of complications and future therapy. Phillip Hench used to say that the arthritic's hand is his "calling card." The patient presents his hand; it is usually warm and moist and the patient flinches as his hand is squeezed. Examination of the joints shows that the involvement is primarily in the proximal interphalangeal joints and metacarpal phalangeal joints. The terminal phalangeal joints are practically never involved in rheumatoid arthritis. Not only are the involved joints tender but they are swollen, and careful palpation reveals synovial thickening. As the disease progresses, there is atrophy of the interossei muscles of the hand, and late in the disease the fingers show a drift to the ulnar side and are associated with subluxation and obvious joint destruction. The wrists are commonly involved and show synovial thickening. The elbows are particularly important to examine for rheumatoid nodules. They are usually on the extensor side. Limitation of shoulder motion is important to note because impairment of shoulder motion makes self-care such as simple daily toilet habits difficult. If the temporomandibular joint is examined with the jaw relaxed, joint capsule swelling may be detected and tenderness indicates the presence of disease. The feet should be examined with the patient standing, because weight-bearing brings out abnormalities such as flat feet; and swelling just below and in front of the malleoli are characteristic of synovial or intra-articular disease and distinguish the swelling from simple peripheral edema. Metatarsal involvement is particularly important to note, because unless the diseased metatarsals are supported and corrected, the patient will experience future difficulty in walking. Examination of the knee and hip is determined by palpation, and in the knee one particularly looks for synovial thickening. If the knee is swollen, this is usually the simplest and easiest joint to tap for examination of joint fluid.[12]

LABORATORY STUDIES

The common significant laboratory abnormalities in rheumatoid arthritis are as follows:

1. <u>Sedimentation rate</u>: This is usually elevated. Occasionally, in a small percentage of cases, the sedimentation rate may be normal at the onset of the disease; but followed over a period of time, the bulk of the cases will show an elevated sedimentation rate.

2. <u>Erythrocyte count, hemoglobin, and hematocrit</u>: Most of the patients will show an anemia, usually normocytic and normochromic and most often in the range of 10 to 11 grams of hemoglobin.

3. <u>White cell count</u>: This is of little diagnostic value. It is usually normal, occasionally slightly elevated. A marked elevation in white blood cell count should alert one to the possibility of an infectious process. A low white blood cell count is associated with systemic lupus, or Felty's syndrome. Marked eosinophilia can be an indication of vasculitis or drug toxicity.

4. <u>Urinalysis</u>: This is usually normal.

5. <u>Chemistry screen</u>: This is seldom of diagnostic value but may show a decrease in total serum protein and a reversal of the albumin globulin ratio. Immunoelectrophoresis may reveal elevations of immunoglobulins: IgM, IgG, and IgA in rheumatoid arthritis.

The diagnosis of rheumatoid arthritis depends upon a history of painful swollen joints, usually bilateral and progressive associated with morning stiffness, usually lasting more than an hour and sometimes the entire day. Fatigue is an important prodromal symptom and accompanies the disease. Physical examination, particularly of the hands and feet will show swelling of the metacarpophalangeal, the proximal interphalangeal, and the metatarsal joints. Swelling of the large joints and synovial thickening are important. The laboratory studies and x-ray changes have been discussed. The presence of a positive antinuclear antibody test in rheumatoid arthritis does not eliminate the diagnosis of rheumatoid arthritis because it occurs in 15 percent of the cases. The absence of a positive RA test does not eliminate the diagnosis of rheumatoid arthritis.

In the differential diagnosis, the following diseases should be considered:

1. Osteoarthritis: This is usually distinguished by its lack of systemic symptoms, the involvement of the terminal phalangeal joints of the hands, the characteristic x-ray changes, and the normal laboratory tests.

2. Rheumatic fever: Rheumatic fever is a disease primarily of young people, and the high ASO titer in rheumatic fever is useful in distinguishing it from rheumatoid arthritis. Patients with rheumatoid arthritis seldom have active manifest carditis as is the case in rheumatic fever. The total absence of progressive joint destruction distinguishes rheumatic fever from rheumatoid arthritis.

3. Polymyalgia rheumatica: This is a disease primarily of older women, characterized by a marked elevation in sedimentation rate and an anemia and the complete absence of any joint swelling. The findings of temporal arteritis on biopsy is diagnostic.

4. Polyarteritis: This is primarily a disease of older males. The presence of eosinophilia and renal involvement should alert one to the possibility. Biopsy or arteriograms are diagnostic.

5. Psoriatic arthritis: Sometimes it is almost impossible to decide whether the patient has psoriatic arthritis or rheumatoid arthritis with psoriasis. Psoriatic arthritis is seronegative. There is involvement of the terminal phalanges, and the late x-ray changes of pencilling and cupping are diagnostic.

6. Ankylosing spondylitis: When there is peripheral joint involvement, this sometimes presents a diagnostic problem. However, ankylosing spondylitis is usually a sero-negative

arthritis affecting younger males. It is HLA-B27 positive and the peripheral joints involved are usually the large joints, the hip, and the knee. In addition, the classic sacroileitis, both clinically and seen on x-ray, is an important distinguishing feature.

7. Reiter's syndrome: This is a disease primarily of young males. The presence of the balanitis circinata and the skin manifestations helps to distinguish the disease from rheumatoid arthritis. However, if the disease becomes chronic and progressive, it is sometimes impossible to distinguish the two.

8. Enteropathic arthritis: Enteropathic arthritis may at times be impossible to distinguish from rheumatoid arthritis, and it is only subsequent events that will establish the diagnosis. If the patient starts with a diagnosed enteropathy, the diagnosis is obvious, but a large percentage of the cases may start with peripheral joint involvement. The clue that the patient may not have a true rheumatoid arthritis is the fact that it is sero-negative and seems to run an atypical course. The diagnosis becomes apparent when the patient develops abdominal symptoms and the diagnosis is established radiologically, by biopsy, and by colonoscopic examination.

9. Systemic lupus erythematosus: For many years, this was confused with rheumatoid arthritis. Until the discovery of the L.E. cell by Hargraves, systemic lupus was seldom diagnosed before the autopsy. Every patient with rheumatoid arthritis should be considered as possibly having systemic lupus, because 70 percent of the patients with systemic lupus initially start with the symptom of arthralgias. The important clues suggesting systemic lupus are a white blood count under 3,000, urine abnormalities, particularly albumin, red cells, white cells, and casts, and blood serum with false positive serology. The presence of L.E. cells is not in itself adequate to make a diagnosis of systemic lupus; and a fluorescent antinuclear antibody test, and an anti-DNA test should also be ordered (see Part Two, Chapter 5, Systemic Lupus Erythematosus).

The treatment of rheumatoid arthritis is to a large extent empirical; and, because of the individual variation in patterns of disease, treatment must be individualized.

Since most physicians learn the disease from a hospital experience where they have seen the chronic progressive nature of the disease, they have a distorted picture of its natural course. In many patients, there may be a natural remission when the disease first starts if not overtreated and if properly handled.[13,14]

Since specific therapy implies the use of toxic drugs and a lifetime of treatment, it is important that when the disease first begins it be treated conservatively. Conservative treatment entails little risk and does not subject the patient to a lifetime of therapy.

Because the patient fears a chronic disease and is in constant pain and because the physician psychologically often needs a cure or dramatic result, conservative therapy is difficult to manage and can be carried out only by a knowledgeable, determined physician.

The first step is patient education.[15] The patient will be buffeted by well-meaning friends, newspaper stories, and concerned relatives. All will offer advice and stories of miraculous recoveries. From the onset it is important that the patient understand the nature of the disease and the danger of miracle cures. This education can be aided by literature obtained from the Arthritis and Rheumatism Foundation, classes for patients, and tape recordings prepared by the physician.

The first step in the conservative approach should be a meeting among the physician, the patient, and the patient's mate. This meeting permits the patient to express his fears and ask questions. It also allows the physician to learn of marital, sexual, economic, or psychological factors that may interfere with a conservative approach.

Where available, the physician should enlist from the very onset the services of the physiotherapist, occupational therapist, and social worker. The physiotherapist helps by teaching the patient passive exercise of disease joints and exercises to prevent deformity. The occupational therapist teaches the patient self-help and provides some of the splinting necessary for joint protection. The social worker explores any emotional and economic problems. An excellent form of physiotherapy is swimming in a warm, heated pool (heated to 85° or 90°). Cooler temperatures cause chilling and muscle spasm and may actually be harmful.

Because of the chronicity of the disease, it is well to discuss the economic problems involved from the onset. The social worker, where available, is invaluable here.

Rest remains the cornerstone of therapy. The rest must be both psychological and physical. It is impossible for a patient to relax and rest at home if burdened with economic pressures, a houseful of screaming children, or an unsympathetic mate. Therefore, before a program of physical rest can begin, the emotional and economic factors must be fully explored and resolved. For some patients, rest may be an impossible goal because of economic or environmental factors.

The optimal amount of physical rest is variable for each patient. The majority of patients with rheumatoid arthritis have fatigue as an accompanying symptom. Because the fatigue may be a prodromal symptom and may be accompanied by minimal laboratory tests, the patient is often suspected of having a functional illness. The object of rest is for the patient to eliminate the fatigue symptom. This concept should be carefully explained. As an analogy, just as chest pain is a deadly symptom for the cardiac patient, so fatigue is a danger signal for the patient with rheumatoid arthritis. In the cardiac patient's case, pain forces him to rest; the arthritic must learn to heed the fatigue signal and to rest as soon as the fatigue appears.

Because of the average patient's need for direction, it is wise to start with a prescribed rest time. My admonition is to sleep as late as possible and to lie down for a rest every afternoon. Under no circumstances should heavy physical labor be undertaken.[16,17]

In addition to physical and emotional rest, rest of an inflamed joint is vital. Use of an inflamed joint is detrimental. Because the rheumatoid joint feels better when in actual use, it is difficult but important to convey to the patient the concept that the use of a diseased joint may be harmful. Total rest of a joint may lead to ankylosis and secondary muscle atrophy which can be prevented by daily passive, nonweight-bearing and nonstressful joint motion. This can be accomplished by the physiotherapist, by instruction in self-physiotherapy, and by swimming in a warm heated pool.[16,17] In select cases, the rest program can best be accomplished in a hospital; in these cases, four weeks of hospitalization at the onset of the disease can be invaluable. Hospitalization provides the patient with an opportunity to be removed from the stresses and strains of daily living and also provides an intensive program of education, physical and occupational therapy, and a modified rest program. It is not desirable for the patient to be at total bed rest while in the hospital.[18,19]

The problem of rest therapy is an empiric one. It is based on long years of clinical experience but is frought with dangers. As

McMahon[20] has wisely pointed out, rest therapy may destroy
motivation and, in susceptible patients, can be used as a psychologic weapon. I recommend Smith's and Polley's article,[16]
with which I am in total agreement.

Because rest cannot be accomplished if the patient is in pain,
drug therapy is essential during this period. The initial drug
of choice is aspirin (see Part One, Chapter 2, The Myth of Aspirin). The patient must be carefully instructed in its use and
advised that, because the aspirin is being taken primarily for
its anti-inflammatory effect, it should be used even if pain is
absent. The patient should also be advised that if problems with
hearing, dizziness, excessive buzzing in the ears, gastrointestinal complaints or allergic reactions develop, the drug should
be discontinued until the physician is contacted. I have seen as
many serious and toxic effects from aspirin as from any of the
other drugs. If aspirin is not tolerated, the newer anti-inflammatory drugs should be used (ibuprofen, fenoprofen, naproxen,
sulindac, and tolmetin). These drugs have an advantage over aspirin in that they do not produce buzzing in the ears or hearing
difficulties and are less prone to cause gastrointestinal upsets.
They have the disadvantage of higher cost. It has been the clinical experience of some physicians[21] that if one of these drugs
does not work, the other might. On a theoretical basis, they
should not be mixed with aspirin; however, most physicians feel
that they are synergistic with aspirin. Since naproxen, fenoprofen, and ibuprofen are from the same drug family, there does
not seem to be any rationale for mixing these three drugs. However, tolmetin is different chemically and it has been suggested
that tolmetin may be synergistic with any of the other three.

Most patients with rheumatoid arthritis do not respond to indomethacin or phenylbutazone, but a small percentage may respond
dramatically to these drugs. If salicylates or the new anti-inflammatory agents are not effective, then it is worth trying first
indomethacin and then phenylbutazone. These drugs should not
be used together, because they have many similar side effects.
The usual dose of indomethacin is 25 mg four times a day, but
dosages as high as 200 mg four times a day may be used. Once
the patient shows a response to indomethacin, then the minimum
maintenance dose should be determined. The usual starting dose
of phenylbutazone is 100 mg four times a day and, again, once
the patient responds, the minimum maintenance dose should be
determined. There is little point in continuing use of these drugs
if the patient does not show a significant response within a few
weeks.

The combination of rest and anti-inflammatory drugs of relatively low toxicity may result in spontaneous remission. Although the results will not be sudden and dramatic, it is worth continuing on this course for at least six months, unless the patient shows signs of deterioration.

DILEMMA

If commencement of more potent therapy is overly delayed, irreversible joint destruction may occur, but if such therapy is started prematurely, it may obscure a spontaneous remission and subject the patient to unnecessary hazards and expense. Once begun, the more potent therapy must be continued for life, because cessation usually results in exacerbation and the drug is seldom as effective the second time.

If the patient is unable to follow a conservative approach for economic or psychologic reasons, if, while on a conservative program, the disease shows relentless progression, or if after a reasonable trial the conservative approach has failed, the patient and the physician should choose among chloroquine, Plaquenil, and gold. My personal choice is for chloroquine. First, there is little risk in taking chloroquine for three months to determine its effectiveness. Secondly, if chloroquine is effective, it will be effective in one or two months, whereas gold requires three to six months to determine its efficacy. Also, chloroquine can be taken orally, whereas gold requires weekly injections and regular laboratory tests. My initial choice for the adult patient is chloroquine, 250 mg to be taken once a day, usually after the evening meal. Before being started on the chloroquine, the patient should be advised of the dangers of retinal toxicity and blindness and should have a baseline examination by an ophthalmologist. The patient should then be seen at regular intervals by the ophthalmologist as long as he is on chloroquine. If chloroquine is successful, results will be apparent in 30 to 90 days. If no objective and subjective results occur within 90 days, there is little point in continuing with the drug. If the drug is effective, it should be maintained for an indefinite period of time. The principle involved is not to exceed one tablet of 250 mg daily and to attempt a reduction in dosage every six months. Thus, at the end of six months, the patient should be started on 250 mg six days out of seven; at the end of a year, on 250 mg five days out of seven; and so forth for an indefinite period until the minimum maintenance dose is found. Complete withdrawal of the drug and subsequent reinitiation if an exacerbation occurs is seldom satisfactory. If the chloroquine is not tolerated, then hydroxychloroquine sulfate (Plaquenil) is substituted. The maximum dose of Plaquenil is 200 mg twice a day. Patients who do not tolerate chloroquine may tolerate the Plaquenil. The same principles apply to the use of Plaquenil as to the use of chloroquine. Results should be expected in 30 to 90 days, regular ophthalmological examinations should be carried out, and the minimum effective dose should be sought if the patient improves.

If chloroquine or Plaquenil are only partially effective or if they fail, gold should be added to the program. I have found gold to be synergistic with chloroquine and Plaquenil. However, if there has been no benefit at all from the chloroquine or Plaquenil, do not continue the drugs. If they have been of benefit objectively and subjectively but the patient is still having active disease, then add gold to the program.

Currently, there are two choices in the United States for gold (see Part One, Chapter 7). I prefer Myochrysine, because it is an aqueous solution as compared to Solganal, which is an oily solution. However, some feel that results are better with Solganal. My advice is to learn to use one or the other well. If the Myochrysine produces nitrinoid reactions, Solganal can be substituted. The usual dosage of gold is weekly injections of 50 mg intramuscularly. However, a dosage as low as 25 mg intramuscularly once a week may prove effective in some cases; there seems to be little benefit in increasing the dosage. The efficacy of gold should be apparent in six months. If it does not work by then there seems to be little benefit in continuing it. However, not all rheumatologists agree; a recent study suggests that the longer gold is continued the better the chances of success. If it succeeds, common experience of a generation of rheumatologists dictates that maintenance on gold therapy of 25 to 50 mg once a month should be continued for life.

In starting gold, the physician should be alert to the fact that it is a toxic drug and deaths are reported almost every year from the use of gold. The patient at each visit should have a complete blood count and urinalysis. The blood smear should be examined by a competent technician to determine that adequate platelets are present, and a platelet count should be done once a month. The commonest toxic manifestation is a dermatitis which may simulate almost any known skin disease. It is usually accompanied by a pruritis. It is wise to ask the patient at each visit if there is itching. Itching is usually the first sign that a pruritus is imminent; and if the gold is withheld, the pruritus may not develop. If a pruritus does develop it is an indication to withhold gold. Continuation of the gold in the presence of a dermatitis can result in serious complications. The dermatitis can be treated with topical corticosteroids, but in severe cases it can be relieved with a short course of oral corticosteroids. If it appears that gold therapy is successful, when the dermatitis clears, a second attempt at gold therapy may be tried and the dermatitis may not reappear. The usual procedure is to give the patient a small test dose, 5-10 mg of gold salt, wait a week and if a dermatitis does not develop, then proceed to a dosage schedule of 25 mg once a week instead of 50 mg once a week. The presence of a marked eosinophilia in the differential blood count may indicate an impending dermatitis and it might be wise to withhold gold if there is a high eosinophilia. When the eosinophilia disappears, an attempt may be made to resume the gold therapy. Albuminuria is a definite contraindication to continuing the gold. Here again, when the albuminuria clears, a second attempt at a lower dosage schedule may be made.

By the third month of gold therapy, there should be some indication as to whether or not the patient is having any benefit. The first indication is often an improvement in the sedimentation rate and a rise in the hemoglobin. If, by six or seven months of therapy, the patient is not responding, it is very unlikely that continuation of the gold therapy will result in a remission. It is important to constantly bear in mind that all kinds of bizarre complications may occur secondary to gold. A stomatitis is not uncommon and may be severe enough to cause malnutrition. Gastrointestinal complaints, diarrhea, and cramps occur. These can be considered minor complications in the sense that they disappear with withholding the drug, and reintroducing the drug at a lower dosage may permit therapy to continue. The major complications are bone marrow depression and if a true bone marrow depression occurs, no further attempts with the drug should be made.

If the accepted methods do not work, then one should consider the newer drugs; a current favorite is penicillamine (Cuprimine Depen), which has recently been approved by the FDA in the treatment of rheumatoid arthritis. The recent admonition of low doses for a long period of time has lessened the incidence of toxicity with penicillamine. In my experience, I have seen patients in whom all other modalities had failed to respond to penicillamine. The high incidence of toxicity associated with penicillamine requires careful monitoring of the drug. At this time it appears that if penicillamine is successful it probably has to be maintained for life. The recent introduction of a 125 mg capsule has permitted finer titration when an attempt is being made to find the minimum effective dose (see Part One, Chapter 8, Penicillamine).

If the patient has not responded to any of the preceding drugs, then one has the choice between immunosuppressives and cortisone. It is rare to find the immunosuppressives used alone.

Therefore, it is probably preferable to start with the cortisone. One should realize that in starting cortisone, one is suppressing symptoms, not altering the course of the disease, and that, once begun, cortisone can seldom be successfully withdrawn.[22] Prednisone is the drug of choice, because it is readily available as an inexpensive generic and can be obtained in 1 and 5 mg tablets. The patient and the pharmacist must be cautioned that it is very difficult to distinguish between the two sizes. The patient is started on a minimal dose of 2 or 3 mg a day. There should not be any rapid changes in dosage; rather, the dosage should be slowly increased until the maximum therapeutic benefit is obtained. The dosage should never exceed 7.5 mg daily in the female or 10 mg daily in the male. Suggestions of alternate day therapy are seldom effective.

When the patient is started on prednisone, the patient should be advised of the long-term, chronic nature of the therapy and that, although it will not alter the course of the disease, it may offer symptomatic relief. The patient should not adjust the dosage of prednisone himself because changes as little as 1 or 2 mg a day may make considerable difference in the way the patient feels. Frequent changes in prednisone may be a factor in prednisone complications. The patient also must be advised that he must never stop prednisone abruptly, as its sudden cessation may be totally incapacitating. The patient should be instructed to carry identification on his person on prednisone, so that the attending physician in an emergency will be aware of the need for supplemental doses of prednisone.

An unresolved question for the physician using long-term prednisone therapy is whether to add empirically to the patient's program prophylactic treatment to prevent peptic ulcer and osteoporosis. This problem has never been resolved scientifically and depends upon the individual physician's personal choice. Some physicians recommend that the patient follow an ambulatory ulcer diet and take antacids regularly after meals and at bedtime. The prevention of osteoporosis is even more empiric. The osteoporosis is probably the consequence of the disease and the steroids. Some physicians recommend the appropriate sex hormone: estrogen in the female and androgen in the male. The question as to whether or not these hormones may be carcinogenic at this time has lessened their popularity in preventing osteoporosis. There are now suggestions that oral calcium and sodium fluoride be used; again at this point in time this program is purely empiric.

Many physicians use the immunosuppressive drugs before starting prednisone. My personal prejudice against them, because of their numerous side effects, has caused me to limit their use to the court of last resort. In my experience, Cytoxan in particular has worked when all the others have failed; however, I dislike using it because of its long-term toxicity. In a desperate situation, where there is complete understanding and permission on the part of the patient, it certainly is worth a trial. Azathioprine is not nearly as toxic as Cytoxan and I would prefer to try Azathioprine before Cytoxan. The major problem is the length of time the patient can wait for a result. The immunosuppressives are usually used in combination with the prednisone and permit a reduction in the dosage of prednisone and occasionally complete withdrawal of the prednisone.

In contemplating withdrawal of the prednisone in a patient with rheumatoid arthritis, project the withdrawal as a slow process taking anywhere from six months to a year. Withdraw the prednisone very slowly in stages and stop the withdrawal if the patient shows an exacerbation. Start by using 1 mg tablets and drop the dosage only 1 mg per day for at least 30 days. Thus, if the patient is on 7 mg of prednisone daily, reduce the dose to 6 mg of prednisone daily and wait 30 days. If the patient shows no exacerbation either clinically or by laboratory tests, then reduce the dose to 5 mg daily and again wait 30 days. The last 5 mg are usually the most difficult to withdraw and one may never succeed in going below this dosage. When the dosage is below 5 mg daily, the drug probably represents a reasonable risk and should not be withdrawn completely.

To this point we have been discussing the ideal patient with rheumatoid arthritis - the patient who has been followed from the onset of the disease. Unfortunately, this does not represent the average patient. Because of the chronicity of the disease, most patients have seen numerous physicians and have had multiple therapy. In treating such a patient, the physician should start from the beginning by evaluating the patient completely and reconfirming the diagnosis. Even the most experienced physician and the most prestigious medical institution may have been mistaken in the diagnosis. The patient may have systemic lupus, or chronic gouty arthritis, or scleroderma, and not rheumatoid arthritis.

Once satisfied that the diagnosis is correct, carefully evaluate the joint involvement and complications so that the rehabilitative efforts can be directed in the proper direction.

Even though the disease is now chronic, have a conference with the patient and his mate and re-educate them.

Evaluate all previous medication that the patient has taken and the reasons why these medications were discontinued. If they were discontinued for valid toxic effects such as peptic ulcer, retinopathy, bone marrow depression, or allergic reactions, do not consider reusing them. If the reason for discontinuing them was minor toxic reactions, or poor patient compliance, or improper dosage, then consider trying them once more. Gold, for example, works best in the early stages of the disease but occasionally when used in the chronic stages, the results can be surprising.

In taking over the management of a previously treated patient, do not withdraw previous medications, particularly the corticosteroids, except for a valid reason. The withdrawal should be slow so that the patient is not "jolted."

If the patient with rheumatoid arthritis is not doing well, carefully examine him for a second disease, particularly an underlying infection in the genitourinary system or pulmonary system; consider whether the drugs may have produced a toxic reaction such as a neuritis or myositis which may mimic the rheumatic disease; look carefully for the possibility of a peptic ulcer, as it is a result of prolonged drug use; consider the possibility of overuse of sedation and analgesics with addiction; and carefully explore the psychosomatic problems of the patient and the patient's family relationship.

If the patient is not doing well, do not change treatment abruptly, as the disease is subject to exacerbation and remissions. Sometimes it is wise to "weather the storm" to see if the symptoms will not subside spontaneously without the addition of further toxic drugs.

Some patients doing poorly benefit by a three- to four-week course of hospitalization, which permits a reasonable program of rest, a comprehensive program of physiotherapy, a chance to escape from the stresses of daily living, and an opportunity for the physician to monitor and adjust drug dosage.

In addition to the drugs previously described, many patients with chronic painful diseases take acetaminophen (Tylenol) and/or propoxyphene (Darvon). Acetaminophen is analgesic but not anti-inflammatory. Some patients prefer it because it usually does not cause gastrointestinal distress. Propoxyphene and its combinations may be as analgesic as aspirin and codeine compounds. Unfortunately, its long-term use in patients with chronic disease may lead to habituation.

The sad fact is that in a small percentage of the patients with rheumatoid arthritis, no matter who the physician and what the medicine, the disease is marked by relentless progression.

Intra-articular corticosteroids may be of occasional value in an acute joint involvement in rheumatoid arthritis. The dosage varies with the joint size. Volumes as large as 1 to 2 cc may be injected in the knee, whereas in the metacarpophalangeal joints the volume would seldom exceed 0.1 cc. Repeated joint injections should not be done, because they may permit overuse of an involved joint, they may actually produce joint damage, or they may introduce joint infection, prohibiting later artificial joint replacement.

ACTH is not normally used in the treatment of rheumatoid arthritis. Some physicians may on occasion give injections of 40 units intramuscularly of the long-acting forms to get the patient over the "hump." Its long-term use is not recommended.

Complications of rheumatoid arthritis are rare, but there are more complications from the drugs used than from the disease. The physician must be alert to the fact that complications do occur in a small percentage of patients and it is impossible for the physician to predict in advance which patient will and which patient will not have a complication. Because of the nature of the disease, many of these complications are unrecognized because the patient's complaints of pain, fatigue, anorexia, dyspnea, and fever are usually attributed to the basic underlying disease. What follows then is a summary of these complications:

A moderate anemia is a common accompaniment of rheumatoid arthritis, it is usually normocytic and normochromic but it may be normocytic, hypochromic, and sometimes microcytic.

The anemia does not respond to oral iron. It will respond to parenteral iron, but this should not be used because the repeated injections of parenteral iron that would be needed to maintain a laboratory improvement of the anemia would result in accumulation of iron stores, causing a hemosiderosis, and would not influence the course of the rheumatoid arthritis.

When the anemia is less than 10 grams, or if there is a sudden drop in hemoglobin one should look for complicating factors such as a blood loss anemia, or a hemolytic anemia, or a macrocytic anemia due to deficiencies in folic acid or vitamin B-12.[25-28]

Rheumatoid nodules occur in approximately 20 percent of the patients with rheumatoid arthritis; and when accompanied by a high

rheumatoid factor in the blood they presage a severe disease
with a poor prognosis and the possibility of many extra-articular manifestations. Pathologically the nodule exhibits a central
area of fibrinoid necrosis surrounded by epithelioid cells and
fibrocytes and then lymphocytes, plasma cells, and fibrous tissues. Clinically they are hard to the feel but freely movable.
They usually occur over the pressure areas, particularly the elbows, around the tendon sheaths of the fingers, at the tendon insertions at the patella, over the buttocks, and in the feet. They
may occur, however, in any of the organs. When they involve
the heart, lung, or the brain they may lead to serious complications. When they occur in the lung they may be mistaken for a
malignancy even when biopsied.

There is no satisfactory treatment for these nodules. The patient should be advised to avoid pressure points. Removal of
the nodules usually results in recurrence. However, where they
are exceedingly painful and under constant pressure, such as in
the feet, an attempt at removal may be tried; but the patient
should be warned that the success rate is low.[29,30]

When rheumatoid arthritis is accompanied by splenomegaly and
leukopenia, the syndrome is called Felty's syndrome after the
man who described it in 1924. It is an unusual manifestation occurring only once in every one or two hundred patients. The
splenomegaly associated with this syndrome does not necessarily
imply a huge spleen; the spleen may be only moderately enlarged.
The hallmark of the disease is granulocytopenia; the count is
usually in the 1-2,000 range, the white blood count may actually
be as low as 500-600 per cubic millimeter. When it is this low,
it is often associated with recurrent bacterial infections which
may manifest themselves as oropharyngeal ulcerations, anal and
perirectal infections, cellulitis and lymphangitis, leg ulcers,
pneumonia, and septicemia.

The bone marrow in patients with this syndrome usually shows
a hyperplastic picture with a maturation arrest of the granulo-
cyte series.

The treatment of Felty's syndrome is a difficult problem, because although the findings may appear ominous, the disease can
pursue a relatively benign course, and natural remissions may
occur without therapeutic interference. The general belief is
that splenectomy may be beneficial in some patients. Splenectomy is usually followed by an improvement in the neutropenia,
a reduction of infections, and a healing of leg ulcers; but later
on there may be a relapse of the neutropenia, and again the patient becomes susceptible to infections. At times the patient does

not respond to splenectomy. Because of the limited experience in the treatment of Felty's syndrome, it is probably wise not to do a splenectomy for neutropenia alone or for a moderate degree of an anemia. The presence of recurrent severe infections and refractory leg ulcers might be considered an indication for splenectomy. There have been reports that lithium carbonate may be of benefit, [31-35] and there have been some reports that long-term testosterone therapy in men would be of benefit. [36] It is still too early to draw any conclusions as to the long-term significance of the reports of the use of these drugs.

Sjogren's syndrome occurs as a complication of rheumatoid arthritis but may be associated with many other of the "autoimmune" diseases (see Part Two, Chapter 18, Sjogren's Syndrome). The treatment of Sjogren's Syndrome is symptomatic. The patient should be monitored for secondary infections, particularly of the eye and of the salivary glands, and for the possibility of renal involvement.

Amyloidosis (see Part Two, Chapter 20, Amyloidosis) - Deposition of amyloid in various organs may be secondary to chronic inflammatory processes. It is a rare complication. The symptoms vary, depending upon the organ involved. The commonest organ involved is the kidney, and proteinuria is the finding that should alert the clinician to the possibility of amyloidosis. Diagnosis is usually made by direct organ or rectal biopsy. There is no proven treatment.

Osteoporosis is a common accompaniment of rheumatoid arthritis. Whether it is a result of disuse, a change in protein metabolism, or is secondary to the drugs used in treatment is a debatable question. The symptoms of osteoporosis usually present themselves as a spontaneous fracture, most frequently involving the dorsal or lumbar vertebrae. Typically, a patient will complain of severe back pain that came on abruptly with no specific history of injury. Diagnosis is made by radiograph. Treatment during the acute phase consists of analgesics and bed rest. Normal mobility should be resumed as soon as possible because disuse may lead to progression of osteoporosis. Therapy is debatable and nonspecific. Androgens, estrogens, vitamin D, and calcium have all been recommended. None is universally accepted. [37]

Rheumatoid heart disease is seldom clinically evident. For a long time it was believed that no greater incidence of heart disease occurred in patients with rheumatoid arthritis than in the general population. [38,39] However, as our diagnostic methods have improved, it has been recognized that patients with rheumatoid arthritis have an increased incidence of myocardial disease and valvular abnormalities. Autopsy studies have regularly demonstrated a large number of heart lesions in patients with rheumatoid arthritis.[40,41] Coronary artery disease occurs in patients with rheumatoid arthritis in about the same incidence that it occurs in the general population.[42] The heart in the rheumatoid may suffer from granulomas, lymphocytic infiltration, constrictive pericarditis, focal myocarditis, and endocarditis.[43]

Treatment of rheumatoid carditis is nonspecific and differs little from that of other cardiopathies. For example, successful aortic valve replacement in a case of rheumatoid carditis has been reported.[44]

Pericarditis, formerly seldom diagnosed in rheumatoid arthritic patients, was considered a rare complication.[45] Although not detectable on the ECG or chest x-ray, pericardial effusion has now been shown by modern echocardiographic studies to be a complication in as high as 44 percent of patients with rheumatoid arthritis. On rare occasions, the pericarditis may precede the onset of clinical rheumatoid arthritis.[47] Over half the patients with pericarditis present no clinical symptoms. The diagnosis is frequently missed; even when chest pain is present, it may be misinterpreted as being secondary to joint or cartilage disease. Occasionally the patient may have a mild fever with the pericarditis. The principal diagnostic sign is the friction rub which may on occasion last for years. It usually has only a systolic component; the diastolic component is unusual. The electrocardiographic changes may be absent or may show the classical configuration of ST elevation with later T wave changes, but usually the less specific changes of generalized T wave inversion or flattening occurs. The evolution of these ECG changes helps to determine whether the disease is a pericarditis, or myocarditis, or coronary insufficiency.[48]

Pericardial effusions probably accompany all cases of pericarditis but they are usually so small that they are seldom detected. They may, however, on rare occasions be severe enough to produce cardiac tamponade or constriction and thus become a serious complication.[49] The diagnosis is frequently missed or delayed. Therefore, congestive heart failure in the patient with rheumatoid arthritis should always be viewed with suspicion. The most helpful diagnostic signs are radiographic evidence of cardiomegaly, associated pleural effusion, pulsus paradoxus, low voltage of the QRS complexes in the ECG. Echo cardiography is helpful in demonstrating the fluid between the parietal and visceral pericardium.[48]

There is no treatment for simple uncomplicated pericarditis and the disease is usually self-limiting. Systemic steroids do not help. Pericardial effusion severe enough to cause acute tamponade is a serious complication and should be treated by pericardiocentesis. If repeated taps are necessary, then a pericardectomy should be done. The operation is very successful.[49] Although cardiac disease is a frequent cause of death in rheumatoid arthritis,[50] it is seldom diagnosed clinically. This is understandable. Chest pain or edema is easily attributed to joint disease; and dyspnea with exertion and angina pectoris are seldom provoked in the patient with rheumatoid arthritis because of their limited physical activity. With the demonstration that cardiac surgery, particularly valvular replacement and pericardectomy, may be of considerable value in these patients, it has become increasingly important to maintain a high degree of suspicion of possible cardiac disease in these patients.

Pleurisy with effusion is the commonest manifestation of rheumatoid lung disease. There may be small amounts of fluid or overwhelming amounts of fluid; usually the effusion is associated with joint disease but in a few rare cases may precede the development of the joint disease. These pleural effusions are serous exudates resembling synovial fluid. The white blood count in the effusion is usually in the area of 5,000 and, peculiarly, often this fluid may exhibit a low glucose content in the absence of any infection.[51] There is a wide range of lung disorders in patients with rheumatoid arthritis. It is impossible to say how many of these are specific associations, how many are due to the debilitated condition of the patient, permitting secondary infections, and how many of them may be related to therapy, particularly steroids, immunosuppressants, gold, and penicillamine.[52,53] A diffuse pulmonary fibrosis, called fibrosing alveolitis, has been described, as well as pulmonary nodules pathologically resembling rheumatoid nodules found elsewhere in the body.[53] The presence of intrapulmonary nodules in coal miners with rheumatoid arthritis was first reported by Caplan, and the disease bears his name. Similar lesions, however, have been described in workers with other inorganic dusts including silica and asbestos.[54-56]

The diagnosis of pulmonary rheumatic disease is made by chest roentgenogram, aspiration, and examination of pleural effusions, bronchoscopy, and lung biopsy. Be alert to the possibility that the lung biopsy may be misinterpreted as being malignant.

The treatment of these complications is very unsatisfactory. There are conflicting reports suggesting that steroids may be of no help, may actually make the condition worse, or may be of benefit in a minority of cases. Other treatments have been immunosuppressive agents and penicillamine. Thus far there is no scientific proof of the efficacy of any specific treatment.[53]

It would seem that the best way to manage the pulmonary complications is to treat the systemic aspects of the disease. The patient should be carefully evaluated for toxic exposures to irritating dusts and secondary invaders such as tuberculosis. One must seriously consider whether the therapy such as gold, penicillamine, or the immunosuppressives are in themselves responsible for the complications.

The eye is so commonly involved in rheumatoid arthritis, either due to the disease itself or to the drugs, that it is well to involve an ophthalmologist in the care of the patient from the very beginning. Iridocyclitis occurs in about 11 percent of patients with juvenile polyarthritis[51] and may be asymptomatic. Therefore, the juvenile polyarthritic must have ophthalmological examinations at regular intervals. Keratoconjunctivitis sicca can cause severe symptoms and may be the cause of severe corneal disease (see Part Two, Chapter 18, Sjogren's Syndrome). An ophthalmologist, in difficult cases, can make the diagnosis with slit lamp examination, the use of the Schirmer's test, and by rose bengal stains of the cornea and conjunctiva. The condition can be treated with artificial tears and in severe cases by obstruction of the lower tear ducts.

Episcleritis may occur and appears to be self-limiting. Scleritis may be particularly severe.[58]

A number of the drugs used in the treatment of rheumatic diseases can cause ocular damage. This includes indomethacin, ibuprofen, cortisone, gold, and chloroquine.[58] Some of these drugs and their complications are as follows:

There is an increased incidence of cataracts and glaucoma associated with the prolonged use of corticosteroids.

Chloroquine and hydroxychloroquine, as discussed in the chapter on these drugs, may lead to serious irreversible retinopathy. In addition, corneal infiltration may occur but is usually reversible. In my personal experience, when we were formerly using much larger doses of these drugs, some patients developed diplopia secondary to a third-nerve palsy. This was quickly reversible with withdrawal of therapy.

Aspirin rarely causes complications but there have been rare reports of allergic kerotitis and conjunctivitis.[59]

Indomethacin has been reported to cause corneal deposits, blurred vision, constricted visual fields, night blindness, and pigment in the fundus. These effects seem to be reversible.[60]

Phenylbutazone has been reported to cause blurred vision, which is reversible.

Ibuprofen has been reported to cause reversible visual changes.

A generalized gold reaction may include blepharitis, conjunctivitis, keratitis, corneal ulcers, and iritis, all of which disappear with cessation of therapy.[61,58]

As is true of so many of the extra-articular manifestations of arthritis, rheumatoid vasculitis is very rarely recognized clinically, but is very commonly found at autopsy.[62]

In 1963 Biwaters and Scott reported a clinical syndrome in rheumatoid arthritis in which there is gangrene of the tips of some of the fingers. They also described splinter hemorrhages due to infarctions at the cuticle of the nail. These occurrences are rare and tend to be self-limiting.[63]

A rare form of generalized vasculitis, associated with rheumatoid arthritis and indistinguishable from polyarteritis except for its pathology, has been identified. The complication seems to occur in steroid-treated patients with active disease in whom steroid reduction has been too rapid or changes in steroid dosage have been too frequent. It may manifest itself with fever, peripheral neuropathy, localized purpura, cutaneous ulcerations, and distal gangrene of an extremity. Fatal complications are rare, but myocardial infarction, gastrointestinal hemorrhage, and intestinal perforation have all been reported as a consequence of arteritis.[62]

Most patients with vasculitis have a benign, self-limiting course and many rheumatologists elect not to treat. In the patient where a severe generalized vasculitis follows a rapid withdrawal of corticosteroids, it would appear logical to resume the steroid medication and then begin a very slow withdrawal at a later date. Immunosuppressives have been reported to be effective, and penicillamine has been used successfully.[64,65]

Neuropathy is a more common complication of rheumatoid arthritis than is usually realized. It may occur as a result of nerve entrapment, secondary to adjacent joint and muscle involvement. It may be secondary to the arteritis. It may be idiopathic or the consequence of drugs used in the treatment of the disease (gold and penicillamine). It is my clinical impression that the diagnosis of peripheral neuropathy is frequently missed because its symptoms are so similar to those of rheumatoid arthritis - muscle pain and muscle weakness. It has been my experience that when the disease is suspected and competent neurological help is sought, objective evidence of neuritis may be found.

Leg ulcers do occur in rheumatoid arthritis and, although infrequent, can be troublesome. They may be secondary to a vasculitis, or they may follow minimal trauma, particularly in a patient on steroids. They may be secondary to impaired circulation caused by the edema commonly associated with rheumatoid arthritis, or they may be idiopathic.[66] The literature lacks information on the treatment of these ulcers, which can be chronic and indolent. I have had reasonable success in treating patients with chronic and indolent ulcers with bed rest with the leg elevated, usually in the hospital, cleaning the ulcer twice a day with a hydrogen peroxide solution and then applying an antibiotic powder, usually a combination of polymyxin B sulfate, zinc bacitracin, and neomycin sulfate (Neosporin). Where there is a great deal of necrotic tissue, the addition of a debriding ointment (collagenase) applied twice a day directly to the lesion is helpful.

PROBLEMS ASSOCIATED WITH SPECIFIC JOINT INVOLVEMENT IN RHEUMATOID ARTHRITIS

Although rheumatoid arthritis seldom involves other parts of the spine, it has an incidence of cervical spine involvement which has been reported to be as high as 40 percent.[67]

Anatomically, the skull rests on the atlas, and the atlas rests on the axis. The axis has a process which projects superiorly called the odontoid process, and the skull pivots at the atlantoaxial joint with the point of rotation being around the odontoid process. Normally, the atlantoaxial joint has a great breadth of movement and is guided by ligaments which protect the spinal cord posteriorly to the odontoid. The odontoid forms a synovial joint anteriorly with the anterior arch of the atlas and posteriorly with the transverse ligaments. These synovial joints may be involved in rheumatoid arthritis, and the transverse ligaments may also be involved and damaged. Involvement of these structures may lead to subluxation of the atlantoaxial joint, with damage to the cervical spinal cord and the vertebral column. Clinical symptoms referable to the cervical spine usually precede radiologic changes. Manifestations vary from no symptoms at all to severe headache, neck pain, arm and leg pain, paresthesias, weakness of both upper and lower extremities, loss of deep tendon reflexes, quadriceps, muscle atrophy, and death. Pain is the most frequent symptom and is usually deep and persistent.[68] A group of patients have described transient but dramatic episodes of quadriplegia of several hours' duration and some complained of blackouts, visual changes, dysarthria, ataxia, and vertigo. These may be secondary to compromised vertebral arteries.

The diagnosis of the condition is usually made by radiographs. Standard AP views of the cervical spine are not diagnostic. Specifically, one should order lateral views of the cervical spine taken in the neutral and forward flexed position. In a forward flexed position, atlanto-odontoid separation greater than 3 mm is diagnostic. The diagnosis can be even more precise with the use of lateral tomograms.

Management is usually conservative. This consists of the use of a cervical collar to prevent forward flexion, since subluxation is maximized in forward flexion. Total immobilization of the cervical spine is not considered necessary. The patients are usually advised to wear their collars day and night, but, if they prefer to sleep without a collar, they are advised not to use a pillow. Cervical traction and neck exercises should be avoided. In a few rare instances, surgical stabilization must be considered, particularly in those patients that develop spinal cord or vertebral artery compression. In many symptomatic patients, studies have shown that subluxation usually stabilizes and may even improve. Generally, all patients with rheumatoid arthritis should have cervical spine films prior to general anesthesia because of flexion and extension of the neck during intubation.

The temporal mandibular joint is occasionally involved in rheumatoid arthritis. The treatment involves the help of a dentist or an oral surgeon. Occasionally, with the jaw relaxed, one can actually palpate swelling of the temporal mandibular joint. A small local injection of insoluble steroids may give temporary relief, but should not be repeated indefinitely. Temporary relief can also be obtained with analgesics, anti-inflammatory agents, hot wet packs, and ultrasound. The best results are obtained with correction of bite. The abnormal bite may be a factor in the development of the disease. Where not a factor in the development of the disease, progression of the temporo-mandibular arthritis leads to an abnormal bite and a great deal of surrounding muscle spasm, thus continuing a vicious circle.[69]

The cricoarytenoid joint is a true synovial articulation. Although rarely involved in rheumatoid arthritis, the joint is occasionally involved and may manifest itself with laryngeal stridor and actually be a life threatening medical emergency demanding an immediate tracheotomy.[70]

In the few patients I have seen with cricoarytenoid joint involvement, the disease has manifested itself first by dyspnea which simulated bronchial asthma and then by hoarseness and nocturnal stridor.

The patient with rheumatoid arthritis who complains of throat symptoms, dysphagia, recurrent sore throats, or difficulty in speech should be examined by an otolaryngologist. Indirect laryngoscopy may reveal changes in the vocal chords. Usually, no specific treatment is indicated for this condition, but a few patients will require a permanent tracheostomy.

Involvement of the shoulder joint is particularly troublesome, because, if permitted to remain unchecked, it will interfere with the patient's self-toilet. When the shoulder joints are involved, intra-articular steroids usually in the neighborhood of about 1/2 cc are temporarily helpful. If the involvement continues and is not responding to the systemic treatment of the disease, I encourage these patients to continue working with a professional physiotherapist in hopes of preventing future difficulties.

Involvement of the elbow, if left untreated, results in flexion contractors. Here too, intra-articular steroids coupled with extensive physiotherapy may be used in acute phases. Involvement of the elbows may be severe enough to involve adjacent nerves and may manifest itself with parasthesias of the fingers and weakness of the hand. The neurologist may be of help here with EMG studies. Treatment consists of synovectomy and nerve transposition. Whenever a patient with involvement of the elbow complains of paresthesias or weakness of the hand, he should be carefully examined, because early surgical treatment prevents later disability.

Involvement of the wrist may lead to median nerve compression (carpal tunnel syndrome). This is a common complication, and the carpal tunnel syndrome may in some cases actually precede the full-blown development of rheumatoid arthritis. The patient characteristically complains of pain in the fingers, usually along the course of the distribution of the median nerve of the hand. The symptoms are much worse at night and may be so severe that the patient has to get out of bed and move the hands to obtain relief. Clinically, once the diagnosis is suspected, pressure or tapping over the carpal tunnel may elicit pain or paresthesia (Tinel's sign). Another excellent test is to have the patient flex the wrist together for a minute, and this may produce pain. In borderline cases, the neurologist using the EMG is diagnostic. Most patients with carpal tunnel syndrome will respond to conservative management. This should consist of splints which place the hand in mild dorsiflexion. The splints can be ordered from most surgical supply stores and properly fitted. Wearing the splints for a month or two at night may be adequate to obtain relief. Where this is not successful, surgery should be done.

Impaired hand function is found in approximately one quarter of the patients with rheumatoid arthritis. The disease frequently starts in the small joints of the hands. It is particularly frustrating to observe a patient who is responding well to systemic therapy such as gold and in whom all clinical evidence of the disease is disappearing continue to suffer from progressive hand deformity. Surgical correction of hand deformity is only minimally successful. Therefore, all that can possibly be done short of surgery to preserve function is worth the effort. The general principle of treatment is to avoid overuse of involved hands and to strengthen the muscles normally used. The occupational therapist has become involved in this problem and is of immeasurable help. Where there is hand involvement, the patient should be referred to the occupational therapist for instructions in hand care and hand preservation. This will consist of splinting of involved joints and of the wrist when it is involved. The splints are usually worn only at night. The patient will also be taught how to minimize stress on the joints while using the hand.[70]

Involvement of the hips, although not common, is a serious complication, because, once started, it usually is relentless in its progress. The physician should be alerted by the patient's complaint of hip pain. Often the initial radiographs may appear normal, particularly when an aseptic necrosis is developing or when there is a fine hairline fracture. It is wise to repeat x-rays in one or two weeks if the pain persists. Sometimes the second film may show pathology missed on the initial examination.

The ideal treatment of hip involvement would be total hospital rest coupled with an active program of physiotherapy for a long period of time. I have never seen this tried and do not imagine that it is practical. The use of crutches to relieve some of the pressure on the hip has been suggested, but the use of crutches in a rheumatoid places potentially harmful pressure on the shoulders. If there is good hand function in the opposing side, a cane will offer the hip considerable relief. Although I seldom use indomethacin or phenylbutazone in rheumatoid arthritis, there have been reports that, when there is hip involvement, these drugs may be particularly effective. In patients on steroid therapy, aseptic necrosis of the femoral head does occur. I have seen it in patients with rheumatoid arthritis who have never had steroids.

The ultimate treatment, aside from the systemic treatment of the disease and the use of analgesics, is total hip replacement (see Part Three, Chapter 6, Surgery in Arthritis). When indicated, the results are usually satisfactory.

Involvement of the knee, like the hip, is a serious complication. I do not favor intra-articular steroid injection more than once or twice. Repeated injections may lead to overuse of the joint and more rapid destruction of the cartilage and may introduce a latent infection which may prevent subsequent surgery. To protect the knee, I usually advise wearing an elastic knee support with hinged metal sides and carrying a cane in the opposite hand. The therapist is particularly effective in teaching the patient to preserve quadriceps muscle function. I do not recommend synovectomy except in the unusual case where the systemic effects of the disease appear to be controlled and the disease tends to linger and be limited to only one knee. Total knee replacement is not as effective as total hip replacement because of its greater incidence of failure. It should not be recommended unless there are no other reasonable alternatives When the knee effusion accumulates posteriorly and ruptures or dissects through the capsule, it produces a condition known as Baker's cyst. The patient presents with a posterior swelling of the knee. If this swelling dissects away from its usual position, it may simulate a thrombophlebitis and in such cases may be indistinguishable except by x-rays (arthrography and venography).

In my experience, aspiration of the joint fluid from the cyst and steroid injections is worthwhile. Many of these people respond to conservative therapy of rest, analgesics, and a few steroid injections. A few require a surgical approach.

When the ankle is involved, I usually recommend an elastic ankle support with stays. This is satisfactory for some patients.

Involvement of the feet and metatarsals is a difficult problem. It is important that properly fitting shoes with a low heel be worn. If there is metatarsal involvement, transverse bars, small strips of leather fitted to the shoe just behind the transverse arch, are helpful. It does take a skilled shoemaker to place these properly. Painful heels can be treated by foam rubber pads inserted in the shoes.

QUESTIONS THAT PATIENTS WITH RHEUMATOID ARTHRITIS USUALLY ASK

Almost every patient with rheumatoid arthritis during the course of the disease will invariably ask questions. Some of these questions and my usual replies are:

1. What about diet and the disease? In my experience, I have yet to have a patient fail to ask this question. When I first started to treat the disease, the only textbook available detailed a number of diets of value in the treatment of rheumatoid arthritis. In 40 years of experience, I have never seen one of these diets work. Dietary fads almost become a religion with some patients and I have found argument futile. Some patients will insist that orange juice makes their disease worse; others will insist that it helps. One recommends bee honey, another gelatin, and yet another alfalfa tea. The correct diet maintains a normal weight and meets normal nutritional requirements.

2. What about vitamins? Fortunes have been made selling vitamins to patients with rheumatoid arthritis. Large doses of vitamin D enjoyed great popularity, until it was discovered that overdosage resulted in renal stones and death. The average American diet contains a normal amount of vitamins. Overdosage simply results in excretion. It is better to spend the money for a pleasant evening out than for the vitamins. I know of no patient with rheumatoid arthritis who has ever been cured with vitamin supplements.

3. Contraception and the pill? The objections to contraceptive pills are the same as those that apply to the general population. At one time it was believed that the patient with rheumatoid arthritis, an autoimmune disease, might be at greater risk in taking the pill than the general population. There have been some reports recently, however, that contraceptive pills may actually offer some protective value in rheumatoid arthritis.

4. Sex? There is no contraindication to normal sexual relations in rheumatoid arthritis, although the disease-associated pain and fatigue may dampen sexual desire and anatomic deformities may make sexual relations more difficult.

In female patients with hand impairment, it is more difficult to properly toilet themselves, and bladder and vaginal
infections may be a common complication. Patients with
rheumatoid arthritis should be told that they are normal
sexually, and their problems should be handled on an individual basis.

5. Pregnancy? This is a difficult question. Most patients with
rheumatoid arthritis are in the childbearing age. At this
time, my general advice is that there is no specific contraindication to pregnancy. During pregnancy, most patients
with rheumatoid arthritis actually have a remission of their
disease. The danger period is postpartum. It is my custom to advise these patients that rest is very important and
that, as pregnancy produces a stress upon the body which is
further aggravated by the birth and care of the child, it is
important to plan to have outside help for at least the first
six months postpartum. During pregnancy, because of the
unknown possibilities of fetal abnormalities, I recommend
discontinuing all drugs. Postpartum, if the mother nurses,
one must consider the effect of the drugs on the mother's
milk. I do not consider rheumatoid arthritis a medical indication for abortion.

6. Work? This is another difficult question which must be decided on an individual basis. A patient who awakens in the
morning with prolonged morning stiffness may have a difficult time meeting a set schedule. Furthermore, these patients are more prone to fatigue than the normal patients.
During acute phases of the disease, the patient is much better off not working and not meeting a schedule of household
duties. On the other hand, in some patients, the psychologic need to work, whether motivated by income or escape
from a home situation, outweighs all other considerations.
In an ideal situation, particularly during acute phases of the
disease, I would prefer that the patient not work and that he
adhere to a regular rest schedule. This advice must be
modified, however, to meet the patient's psychologic and
economic needs.

7. Spa therapy and vacations? The use of spas dates to ancient
Roman times and to specific cities in the Roman Empire.
Carlsbad and Bath were both set aside for these patients.
Any patient with a chronic disease feels better with a change
of environment, good food, rest, fresh air, and a little
pampering.

8. Exercise? A moderate amount of exercise is necessary to maintain body and muscle tone, but improper exercise and use of an acutely involved joint is damaging. The patient should not exercise to the point of fatigue, and an acutely involved joint should be exercised only passively. The fact that a joint may feel better while being used does not indicate that it is being helped. The test is persistence of pain after use, with persistence indicating overuse. Swimming in a warm heated pool is a good form of exercise, because it permits use of joints without putting weight on them. The pool should be heated to over 80°. A cooler pool results in muscle spasm and hinders rather than helps.

9. The relationship of the job to rheumatoid arthritis? I have never known a particular occupation or injury to cause this disease. A direct injury to a joint, however, may occasionally precipitate an involvement of that specific joint when the disease is systemically active.

10. Travel? There is no contraindication to travel, provided it is not stressful and adequate rest periods are provided. When the patient is on a specific regular medication such as gold, missing one or two injections should not be harmful. When the patient is on a regular dosage schedule and will be absent for a long period of time, a letter describing his illness and the gold dosage schedule will usually enable him to obtain an appropriate injection at another physician's office or hospital emergency room.

11. Acetaminophen (Tylenol, etc.)? There is no contraindicato these drugs. They do provide pain relief but are not anti-inflammatory. They are less prone to cause gastrointestinal upsets than the salicylates or other anti-inflammatory agents.

12. The advice of well-meaning friends about miracle cures in foreign countries? Usually these physicians, unbeknownst to the patient, use some form of corticosteroids. Even when they insist that no corticosteroids are present in their medication, one cannot interpret the quick relief other than by the use of corticosteroids.

13. The announcement every three months in some sections of the press of new and miraculous cures? If a person had a cure for rheumatoid arthritis that would stand the test of time and scrutiny by his peers, he would be given a Nobel prize. He would have economic security and would be

recognized for perpetuity. Why would he announce it to the press and not to his peers?

14. Is there a cure? There is no known cure for the disease. A few fortunate patients will go into a spontaneous remission, particularly at the onset of the disease. Another larger group may obtain almost the equivalent of a spontaneous remission with some of the drugs, but in a few patients, no matter what is done, the disease will relentlessly progress.

15. What about the suggestion that cod liver oil, taken by mouth, gets into the blood stream and lubricates the joints? This is as valid as the theory of one of my patients who insists that she is able to get around only by spraying a lubricant on her joints.

16. What about moving to a warm, dry climate? I once had a secretary who decided to marry one of my patients with rheumatoid arthritis. My treatment had been a failure and she was certain that she could rescue him. They sold all their possessions, moved to a warm dry climate, came back a year later - broke - and the arthritis was much worse. His arthritis improved when they settled and developed a successful business. It is not the climate as much as the atmospheric pressure which seems to affect patients with rheumatoid arthritis. The right place to live is where the patient is most secure economically and happiest. There is no specific advantage to changing climate.

SUMMARY

Rheumatoid arthritis is primarily a disease of young women, but it occurs in every age group and in both sexes. It usually starts as a bilateral symmetrical involvement of the peripheral joints characterized by pain, stiffness, and swelling. It tends to be chronic and progressive. It may, however, start as a monoarticular disease and it may also start with exacerbations and remissions. It is a systemic disease associated with systemic symptoms: fever, fatigue, anorexia, and prolonged morning stiffness. Laboratory tests may be normal at the onset of the disease but an anemia and an elevated sedimentation rate are frequent and common accompaniments. The so-called RA test is an agglutination test and is positive in 70 percent of the cases, but a negative RA test does not rule out the diagnosis, nor does a positive RA test by itself make the diagnosis. X-ray changes occur only as the disease progresses, and therefore, at the initial onset of the disease, the radiograph is often interpreted as being normal. Systemic lupus erythematosus may mimic rheumatoid arthritis, and every case of rheumatoid arthritis should be suspect as possibly being systemic lupus. Rheumatoid arthritis is not limited to the joints alone; the pathology may involve tendons, muscles, and ligaments. Twenty percent of the cases have hard peripheral subcutaneous nodules which usually develop at points of stress. Although other organ systems are rarely involved, these complications do occur and manifest themselves as pericarditis, carditis, pleuritis, neuritis, myositis, osteoporosis, leukopenia, uveitis, arteritis, and peripheral neuritis. Renal involvement is rare.

Because many of the cases in their initial onset may, if not overtreated, go into a total remission, it is important that early cases not be overtreated. The initial treatment should be a prescribed program of rest and use of the least toxic, nonsteroidal, anti-inflammatory agents: aspirin, ibuprofen, naproxen, fenoprofen, tolmetin, sulindac. A few cases may respond to indomethacin or phenylbutazone.

If a conservative approach is not effective, then the choice lies between antimalarials (chloroquine or Plaquenil) or gold. My own personal preference is to try the antimalarials first, but because of serious retinal toxicity, some authorities would bypass the antimalarials. Gold has stood the test of time. The usual dosage is 50 mg once a week until a total of 1,000 mg has been given. It should be monitored by blood counts and urinalysis. If there is no improvement by the time 1,000 mg have been given, there is little point in continuing. If the patient does improve with the gold, then the patient should be on maintenance dosage gold 50 mg once a month for life. Discontinuing the gold frequently results in an exacerbation.

If gold is not successful, the choice lies between penicillamine and the immunosuppressive agents (azathioprine, Cytoxan, Leukeran, methotrexate). The current favorite is penicillamine. The present recommended dosage is an initial starting dose of 250 mg of penicillamine daily for three months and then increments of 250 mg every three months until a satisfactory remission is induced, and then a minimum maintenance dose. The drug, although recently approved by the FDA, is toxic and must be carefully monitored.

In a few cases prednisone is the only drug that works. The minimum effective dose should be given, and should never exceed 7.5 mg in the female, 10 mg in the male.

The immunosuppressives may work when all else fails. Their toxicity remains a serious problem.

REFERENCES

1. Duthie, J.J.: Rheumatoid Arthritis. Textbook of the Rheumatic Diseases. Copeman, W.S.C. (ed.), E & S Livingstone Ltd., Edinburgh, London, and New York, 1969, p. 259.

2. Person, D.A. and Sharp, J.T.: The etiology of rheumatoid arthritis. Bulletin on Rheumatic Diseases 27:888, 1976-77.

3. Christian, L.: Etiology and pathogenesis of rheumatoid arthritis. In: Modern Topics in Rheumatology, Ch. 1, Hughes, G.R.V. (ed.), Year Book Medical Publishers, Chicago, 1976.

4. Phillips, P.E.: Virus infections and rheumatic disease. In: Modern Topics in Rheumatology, Ch. 2, Hughes, G.R.V. (ed.), Year Book Medical Publishers, Chicago, 1976.

5. Selye, H.: General adaptation syndrome and diseases of adaptation. Journal of Clinical Endocrinology 6:117, 1946.

6. Persellin, R.H.: The effect of pregnancy on rheumatoid arthritis. Bulletin on Rheumatic Diseases 27:922, 1976-77.

7. Singer, J.M. and Plotz, C.M.: The latex fixation test. American Journal of Medicine 21:888, 1956.

8. Plotz, C.M. and Singer, J.M.: The latex fixation test. American Journal of Medicine 21:893, 1956.

9. Bartfield, H.: Distribution of rheumatoid factor activity in nonrheumatoid states. Annals of the New York Academy of Science 168:30, 1969.

10. Biundo, J.J. and Cumings, N.A.: Biochemical, hematological and immunological tests. In: Rheumatic Diseases, Katz, W.A., (ed.), J.B. Lippincott Co., Philadelphia, 1977, p. 265.

11. Bywaters, E.G.L.: The early radiological signs of rheumatoid arthritis. Bulletin on Rheumatic Diseases 11:231, 1960.

12. Bilka, P.J.: Physical examination of the arthritic patient. Bulletin on Rheumatic Diseases 20:596, 1970.

13. O'Sullivan, J.B. and Cathcart, E.S.: The prevalence of rheumatoid arthritis. Annals of Internal Medicine 76:573, 1972.

14. Beall, G. and Cobb, S.: The frequency distribution of rheumatoid arthritis as shown by period examinations. Journal of Chronic Diseases 14:291-310, 1961.

15. Kaye, R.L. and Hammond, A.H.: Understanding rheumatoid arthritis: Evaluation of a patient education program. Journal of the American Medical Association 239:2466, 1978.

16. Smith, D. and Polley, H.F.: Rest therapy for rheumatoid arthritis. Mayo Clinic Proceedings 53:141, 1978.

17. Ferguson, R.H.: Rheumatoid arthritis and rest. Mayo Clinic Proceedings 53:195, 1978.

18. Mills, J.A., et al.: Value of bed rest in patients with rheumatoid arthritis. The New England Journal of Medicine 284:453, 1971.

19. Lee, P., et al.: Benefits of hospitalization in rheumatoid arthritis. Quarterly Journal of Medicine 43:205, 1974.

20. McMahon, J.M.: Rest therapy for rheumatoid arthritis. Mayo Clinic Proceedings 53:477, 1978.

21. Ehrlich, G.E.: Nonsteroidal Anti-inflammatory Paper Presented at American Society of Experimental Pharmacology and Therapeutics, Atlanta, GA, March, 1978.

22. Bernsten, C.A. and Freyberg, R.H.: Evaluation of the status of patients with rheumatoid arthritis after five or more years of corticosteroid treatment. Bulletin on Rheumatic Diseases 12:261, 1961.

23. Hahn, T.J.: Corticosteroid-induced osteopenia. Archives of Internal Medicine 138:882, 1978.

24. Katz, W.A.: Rheumatic Diseases. J.B. Lippincott Co., Philadelphia, 1977, p. 431.

25. Jeffry, M.R.: Some observations on anemia in rheumatoid arthritis. Blood 8:502-510, 1953.

26. Partridge, R.E., et al.: Incidence of macrocytic anemia in rheumatoid arthritis. British Medical Journal 1:89, 1963.

27. Gough, K.R., et al.: Folic acid deficiency in rheumatoid arthritis. British Medical Journal 1:212, 1964.

28. Mongan, E.S. and Jalox, R.F.: Erythrocyte survival in rheumatoid arthritis. Arthritis and Rheumatism 7:481, 1964.

29. Subcutaneous rheumatoid nodules (Editorial). British Medical Journal 1:877, 1965.

30. Kellgren, J.H., et al.: Clinical significance of the rheumatoid serum factor. British Medical Journal 1:523, 1959.

31. Felty, A.R.: Chronic arthritis in the adult, associated with splenomegaly and leukopenia: A report of five cases of an unusual clinical syndrome. Bulletin of Johns Hopkins Hospital 35:16, 1924.

32. Louie, J.S. and Pearson, C.M.: Felty's Syndrome. Seminars in Hematology 8:216, 1971.

33. Bennett, R.M.: Hematological changes in rheumatoid arthritis. Clinics in Rheumatic Disease 3:433, 1977.

34. Lothra, H.S. and Hunder, G.G.: Spontaneous remission of Felty's syndrome. Arthritis and Rheumatism 18:515, 1975.

35. Gupta, R.C., et al.: Efficiency of lithium in rheumatoid arthritis with granulocytopenia (Felty's Syndrome). Arthritis and Rheumatism 18:179, 1975.

36. Wimer, B.M. and Sloan M.M.: Remission of Felty's syndrome with long-term testosterone therapy. Journal of the American Medical Association 223:671, 1973.

37. Dent, C.E.: Osteoporosis. Postgraduate Medical Journal (Supplement) 42:583, 1966.

38. Short, C.L., et al.: Rheumatoid Arthritis. Harvard University Press, Cambridge, MA, 1957.

39. Gibberd, F.B.: A survey of four hundred and six cases of rheumatoid arthritis. ACTA Rheumatologica Scandinavica 11:62, 1965.

40. Cathcart, E.S., et al.: Rheumatoid heart disease: A study of the incidence and nature of cardiac lesions in rheumatoid arthritis. The New England Journal of Medicine 266:959, 1962.

41. Baggenstoss, A.H. and Rosenberg, E.F.: Cardiac lesions associated with chronic infectious arthritis. Archives of Internal Medicine 67:241, 1941.

42. Liebowitz, W.B.: The heart in rheumatoid arthritis (rheumatoid disease: A clinical and pathological study of sixty-two cases). Annals of Internal Medicine 58:102, 1963.

43. Sokoloff, L., et al.: Vascular lesions in rheumatoid arthritis. Journal of Chronic Diseases 5:668, 1957.

44. Iveson, J.M.I., et al.: Aortic valve incompetence and replacement in rheumatoid arthritis. Annals of Rheumatic Disease 34:312, 1975.

45. Gordon, D.A., et al.: The extra-articular features of rheumatoid arthritis - A systematic analysis of 127 cases. American Journal of Medicine 54:445, 1973.

46. Nomeir, A.M., et al.: Cardiac involvement in rheumatoid arthritis. Annals of Internal Medicine 79:800, 1973.

47. Grossman, L.A.: Acute pericarditis with subsequent clinical rheumatoid arthritis. Archives of Internal Medicine 109:665, 1962.

48. Iveson, J.M.I., et al.: Cardiac involvement in rheumatoid disease. In: Clinics in Rheumatic Disease. W.B. Saunders Co., Philadelphia, 1977, p. 467.

49. Thadani, V., et al.: Cardiac tamponade, constrictive pericarditis, and pericardial effusion and pericardial resection in rheumatoid arthritis. Medicine 54:261, 1975.

50. Southwood, E.J., et al.: Causes of death in rheumatoid disease. Arthritis and Rheumatism 2:49, 1959.

51. Walker, et al.: Pulmonary lesions and rheumatoid arthritis. Medicine 47:405, 1968.

52. Arnoff, A., et al.: Lung lesions in rheumatoid arthritis. British Medical Journal 2:228, 1955.

53. Turner-Warwick, M.: Pulmonary manifestations of rheumatoid disease. In: Clinics in Rheumatic Disease, W.B. Saunders Co., 1977, p. 549.

54. Caplan, A.: Certain unusual radiological appearances in the chest of coal miners suffering from rheumatoid arthritis. Thorax 8:29, 1953.

55. Hayes, D.S., et al.: A case of Caplan's syndrome in a roof tile maker. Tubercle 41:143, 1960.

56. Telleson, W.G : Rheumatoid pneumonoconiosis (Caplan's syndrome) in asbestos worker. Thorax 16:372, 1961.

57. Smiley, W.K.: The eye in juvenile rheumatoid arthritis. Transactions of the Ophthalmological Societies of the United Kingdom 94:817, 1974.

58. Hazleman, B.L., et al.: Ocular complications of rheumatoid arthritis. In: Clinics in Rheumatic Disease. W.B. Saunders Co., Philadelphia, 1977, p. 501.

59. Grant, W.M.: Toxicology of the Eye. Charles C Thomas Publishers, Springfield, 1962.

60. Burns, C.A.: Indomethacin-reduced retinal sensitivity and corneal deposits. American Journal of Ophthalmology 66: 825, 1968.

61. Goldstein, J.N.: Effect of drugs on cornea, conjunctiva and lids. International Ophthalmology Clinics 11:13, 1971.

62. Kulka, J.P.: The vascular lesions of rheumatoid arthritis. Bulletin on Rheumatic Diseases 10:201, 1959.

63. Bywaters, E.G.L. and Scott, J.L.T.: The natural history of vascular lesions in rheumatoid arthritis. Journal of Chronic Diseases 16:905, 1963.

64. Weisman, M., et al.: Cryoglobulinemia in rheumatoid arthritis: Significance in serum of patients with rheumatoid vasculitis. Journal of Clinical Investigation 56:725, 1975.

65. Jaffe, I.A., et al.: Rheumatoid vasculitis - Report of a second case treated with penicillamine. Arthritis and Rheumatism 11:585, 1968.

66. Wilkinson, M., et al.: Leg ulcers complicating rheumatoid arthritis. Scottish Medical Journal 10:175, 1965.

67. Sharp, J., et al.: Rheumatoid arthritis of the cervical spine in adults. Annals of Rheumatic Disease 17:303, 1958.

68. Bland, J.H.: Rheumatoid arthritis of the cervical spine. Bulletin on Rheumatic Diseases 13:471, 1967.

69. Guralnick, W., et al.: Temporomandibular joint afflictions. The New England Journal of Medicine 299:123, 1978.

70. Vassalo, C.L.: Rheumatoid arthritis of cricoarytenoid joints: Cause of upper airway obstruction. Archives of Internal Medicine 17:273, 1966.

71. Kuhns, J.C.: The preservation of hand function in rheumatoid arthritis. Bulletin on Rheumatic Diseases 10:199, 1959.

CHAPTER 5: SYSTEMIC LUPUS ERYTHEMATOSUS

"The red wolf is gnawing at me."

A patient with systemic lupus erythematosus

There is a bizarre multisystem, multisymptom disease nondescriptly called systemic lupus erythematosus and considered the province of the rheumatologist, although its symptoms, signs, and pathology cross many disciplines. Because different systems are involved in individual patients, treatment must be individualized.

To understand the disease one must follow its historical development. The original term lupus (wolf) described a skin disease characterized by ulcerating lesions of the cheeks and recognized as early as the thirteenth century. The lesions were thought to be due to tuberculosis or cancer. A hundred years ago the rash involving the face was described as being butterfly in appearance because of symmetrical cheek involvement, a description still used today.

By the turn of the century, Osler and others recognized that the skin lesions could be accompanied by systemic symptoms and systemic involvement.[1,2] In 1923 Libman and Sacks noted that some patients with lupus suffered from a form of endocarditis in which there were wart-like vegetations on the cardiac valves but no evidence of bacterial infection.[3] Initially it was assumed that they had described a new disease, but it was soon recognized that many of their patients, in addition to having cardiac symptoms, also had arthralgias, skin rashes, and pulmonary disease. In essence they were describing systemic lupus.[4] By 1935 it was recognized that many of these patients had kidney involvement, and the phrase "wirelooping" came into use to describe the pathology involving the glomeruli. The phrase is still used today in describing some of the pathology seen in renal lupus.[5]

By 1940 a disease which for centuries had been considered primarily a skin disease was now generally recognized as a systemic disease, characterized by various skin rashes but particularly by a butterfly rash of the face and by arthralgias and cardiac and renal involvement. The disease was generally considered fatal.[6]

For all practical purposes the diagnosis was usually made at autopsy. The dermatologist seeing the butterfly rash thought of the disease as a local condition and called it discoid lupus. The cardiologist, in a difficult case of endocarditis with repeated negative blood cultures, would hazard a guess of Libman-Sacks disease, and the rheumatologist following the arthritic patient who had renal disease might consider lupus, but the actual diagnosis was usually made after death.

Our current concept of lupus dates to 1948 when Hargraves described a peculiar leukocyte that he observed in bone marrow. The cell appeared to have ingested its own nucleus or the nucleus of another leukocyte. Hargraves was a hematologist at the Mayo Clinic who delighted in examining bone marrow in difficult diagnostic problems. While studying the marrow in cases that would now be diagnosed as lupus, he described two unusual cells which he named the "tart cell" and the "L.E. cell." He showed true genius with his statement that "these cells represent either a phagocytosis of free nuclear material or the actual autolysis of one or more lobes of the nucleus of the involved cells." On the basis of morphology alone, he predicted what the immunochemist would subsequently prove.[7]

Hargraves originally thought that these cells occurred only in bone marrow. The failure of some investigators to duplicate his findings led him to re-evaluate his technique. In so doing, he realized that it was his practice, after drawing the bone marrow at St. Mary's Hospital in Rochester, Minnesota, to travel a considerable distance to the Mayo Clinic, carrying the sample of the marrow in his breast pocket and thus incubating it. As he extended his studies, it became obvious that the L.E. cell was an in vitro and not an in vivo phenomenon.[8-10] Eventually it was demonstrated that the L.E. cell could also be found in the peripheral blood.

The discovery of the L.E. cell opened a new door for clinicians. What had primarily been a rare disease seldom diagnosed was now on the lips of every medical student. Lupus had arrived! It soon became apparent that the L.E. cell was not a specific diagnostic test, for it was positive in only 60 percent of the proven cases of lupus and false positives were common in such diseases as rheumatoid arthritis, scleroderma, and hepatitis.[11-13]

The nonspecificity of the L.E. cell test led clinicians into eso-
teric discussions as to whether or not the patient had lupus or
had rheumatoid arthritis with L.E. cells. The problem was further complicated by variations in technique and interpretation of
the slides from the peripheral blood and from the bone marrow.
The multiple techniques of slide preparation and the fact that a
patient with proven lupus might have positive cells at one time
and negative cells at another time led to confusion. The test was
helpful, but it was not an answer to the clinician looking for specific diagnostic tests.

The next advance was made by the immunochemists who appreciated that the L.E. cell phenomenon was the result of a factor
in the plasma which reacted with cell nuclei, changing the nuclear material which was then absorbed by the leukocyte. The
factor responsible for the L.E. cell phenomenon could be labeled an antibody and the cell material could be considered an
antigen. It soon became clear that the L.E. cell factor was a
gamma globulin: IgG.[14-16]

The specific nuclear antigen is the basic cell material: DNA.[17]
Immunochemists proved what Hargrave had speculated upon. The
L.E. cell phenomenon was a biological test for the recognition
of circulating antibodies to DNA histone nuclear protein. The
test, however, still could not be used clinically because rigid
physical chemical conditions had to be met before the results
could be interpreted.[18] The next step was the development of
the immunofluorescent technique. In this technique thin tissue
slices, usually animal liver, were treated with fluorescent-la-
beled sera and then examined by ultraviolet light under the microscope for fluorescence. The presence of fluorescence would
indicate that antibodies were present.[19]

It became obvious, as this technique was used by various laboratories, that different patient sera would produce different patterns of nuclear staining and fluorescence. The patterns were
variously described as either being homogeneous, speckled, or
nucleolar. This variation in pattern-staining suggested that antibodies from different patient sera reacted with different parts
of the cell nucleus. It was subsequently shown that this variation
in pattern was due to the antibody reacting to different fractions
such as DNA, singlestranded DNA, native DNA, and treated
DNA.[20]

Antibodies which are specific for at least seven different nuclear
constituents have now been described in patients with lupus. Of
particular interest are the antibodies which are specific for DNA

doublestranded, for these are found almost exclusively in the serum of patients with lupus.[21]

Apparently, SLE is a disease in which there is an antigen antibody interaction: the reaction takes place between an antibody in the patient and an antigen from a cell nucleus native to the patient or possibly a cell nucleus that is altered by an invading virus. An individual patient may have multiple antibodies to various nuclear proteins or may have antibodies which are specific for different organs (thyroid, heart muscle, or kidney).[22,23]

The antinuclear antibodies in themselves have no direct pathologic effect. Antinuclear antibodies cross the placental barrier and are found in the infants of SLE mothers. No known clinical disease occurs in these infants.[24] Apparently, pathology develops only when the antigen antibody reaction .fixes complement and initiates an inflammatory reaction.

Complements are serum proteins and constitute more than 10 percent of the serum globulins. They contain significant amounts of carbohydrates. By international agreement the various components of the complement system are symbolized by a capital C and a number. Thus, C1-C2-C3-C4.[25]

Systemic lupus has been produced by breeding special strains of mice and dogs described as New Zealand mice and dogs. The disease in these animals is similar to systemic lupus in humans, giving us an excellent experimental model. In these animals virus and environmental factors (drugs, chemicals, diet, hormones) can alter the disease;[26,27] so the debate rages as to whether SLE is a genetic disease, a viral disease, or a combination of factors. At this time it appears that it is a multifactoral disease and that different factors may be of varying degrees of importance in different situations.

To summarize, systemic lupus is a multifactoral disease with genetics and viruses playing major roles. An antigen antibody reaction occurs at a variety of body tissues. With the interaction of complement, tissue damage transpires at the sites where immune complexes have been deposited.[28]

The characteristics and prognosis of the disease depend on the organs involved, the most critical organs being the kidney and the brain. In the kidney, at least three pathologic processes are recognized: a focal proliferative form, a diffuse proliferative form, and a membranous form of glomerulonephritis. It is generally believed that the focal proliferative form carries a good prognosis and that the diffuse forms carry a poor prognosis. The classification of pathology is still in a state of flux. It is not yet certain whether various histologies represent separate processes or are simply part of a continuum of process.[29] The natural history of systemic lupus would indicate that the prognosis is good unless there is involvement of the renal or central nervous system.[30]

Lupus has replaced syphilis as a great mimic. It is chameleon in character and a diagnosis may be simple or slippery and elusive. In one patient it appears as an acute psychosis, in another as a pericarditis, and in a third as a nephrosis. It is thought of as a multisystem disease that may remain a single system disease for years before a second organ becomes involved. Any time the clinical picture is bizarre, atypical, or undiagnosed, lupus should be considered in the differential diagnosis. The patients may vary from a neurasthenic young woman complaining of fatigue to a critically ill patient with rash, fever, arthralgia, and nephritis.

Rheumatologists always consider the diagnosis of lupus in all cases of arthralgia. The particular clues in such patients may be a low white blood count, multiple system involvement, abnormalities in the urine, fever, dermatitis, sun sensitivity, and a false positive serology for syphilis. At one time it was thought that patients with lupus arthropathy would not develop joint destruction, but recent reports indicate that up to 30 percent of the patients with lupus may have a deforming and destructive arthritis.[31-33] Lupus is usually considered a disease of young females, but males do develop the disease. All age groups from children to the elderly may be afflicted, and there appears to be a particularly high incidence in black women. Lupus may initially manifest itself as any one of the following:

1. Grand mal seizure
2. Unexplained alopecia
3. Butterfly skin rash
4. Psychosis
5. Unexplained fevers
6. Thrombocytopenia
7. Hemolytic anemia
8. Raynaud's phenomenon
9. Lesions in the mouth
10. Photosensitivity
11. Pericarditis
12. Pleural effusion

13. Endocarditis
14. Leukopenia
15. Nephritis

Lupus is usually a disease of exclusion. One must bear in mind that lupus is not the most common cause of either seizures or skin rashes. It is only when other diseases have been ruled out and there is evidence of multisystem involvement that the diagnosis of lupus becomes apparent. Because of the multiplicity of signs and symptoms, the American Rheumatism Association in 1971 appointed a committee to standardize the diagnosis and to bring order out of the then existing chaos. The committee wisely pointed out that its resulting criteria were only tentative, were subject to change as knowledge developed, and were not meant to supersede the skill of an experienced clinician; they were simply a set of guidelines. Thus, the presence of an antinuclear antibody is not listed in the original criteria, because at the time the criteria were published, the antinuclear antibody and anti-DNA tests had not been standardized.

The preliminary criteria for the classification of SLE as developed by the committee are based on 14 manifestations. It is suggested that the diagnosis of SLE not be made unless at least four or more of the 14 manifestations are present, serially or simultaneously, during any interval of observation. The criteria are as follows:[34]

1. Facial erythema (butterfly rash)
2. Discoid lupus erythematosus, raised patches with adherent keratotic scaling and follicular plugging may be present anywhere on the body.
3. Raynaud's phenomenon
4. Alopecia
5. Photosensitivity
6. Oral or nasal pharyngeal ulceration
7. Arthritis without deformity. One or more peripheral joints involved with any of the following in the absence of deformity:
   a) pain on motion
   b) tenderness
   c) effusion or periarticular soft tissue swelling
8. L.E. cells
9. Chronic false positive serologic test for syphilis (S.T.S.)
10. Profuse proteinuria
11. Cellular casts
12. One or both of the following:
    a) pleuritis
    b) pericarditis

13. One or both of the following:
    a) psychosis
    b) convulsions
14. One or more of the following:
    a) hemolytic anemia
    b) leukopenia (white blood count less than 4,000 per cubic millimeter on two or more occasions
    c) thrombocytopenia platelet count less than 100,000 per cubic millimeter

There has been skepticism over the above criteria from their initial description.[35] One university clinic has reported that in one patient out of four in whom they have made the diagnosis of lupus, the diagnostic criteria have not been met. However, the committee never intended that the criteria be absolute; they were to be used only as guidelines.[36] When we add to these criteria the fluorescent antinuclear antibody test and the anti-DNA test which has recently been developed, a good set of guidelines are present for the average physician.[37]

In 1954 two groups reported a disease in humans resembling lupus but caused by drugs.[38,39] Since this first description of hydralazine - (Apresoline) induced lupus in 1954, numerous other drugs have been implicated in the etiology of the disease. Drugs implicated as activators of systemic lupus include procainamide (Pronestyl), hydralazine (Apresoline), and diphenylhydantoin (Dilantin).

Drug-induced lupus differs from true SLE in that the antinative DNA tests are negative and the disease disappears when the drug is discontinued, although it may take considerable time before all symptoms are gone. Drug-induced lupus resembles true SLE, but renal disease is rare, serum complement levels are never decreased, and the prognosis is good if the drug is discontinued. Although oral contraceptives have been indicted as a cause of drug-induced lupus, their role in the disease has never been proven. Many physicians suggest that women with lupus refrain from taking contraceptive pills, but there is no strong evidence that patients who disregard this advice suffer any ill consequences.[40,41]

THE LABORATORY TESTS

Unfortunately, unlike syphilis where a specific serologic test exists, no such specific test exists for lupus. The L.E. cell test suffers from its lack of specificity, its need for an expert to interpret it, and its false positives. Thus, Dubois, an expert's expert, reports an incidence of 75.7 percent positive L.E. cell preps in patients studied numerous times, over a long period. In one patient with clinically active lupus, 44 L.E. cell tests were performed over a period of ten years before the first positive result was obtained.[42]

The L.E. cell prep has been largely replaced by the newer antinuclear antibody tests. The L.E. cell prep, however, is still a valid test when properly done and properly interpreted. Its advantage is that it can be done in small laboratories with simple equipment and can be rapidly reported. Its major disadvantage is its lack of specificity.

The fluorescent antinuclear antibody test has the disadvantage of being supersensitive. It is unlikely that the patient has lupus if repeated fluorescent antinuclear antibody tests are negative. However, a positive test does not establish a diagnosis of lupus because of its sensitivity. The fluorescent test also has the disadvantage that it can be done only by laboratories with fluorescent microscopes and trained technicians.

A recent development is the anti-DNA test. This is more specific than the fluorescent antibody test and in high titer, it can be used to monitor the response to therapy. The major disadvantage of the test is that it is still not standardized. Titers differ from various laboratories, and the test can be done only in large research-type laboratories. Some recent kits make the technique easier but still require a fluorescent microscope.

Some laboratories now offer serum complement levels either as whole complement, C3-C4, or CH50. Serum complement levels are of no value in making a diagnosis of lupus, but a low serum complement level may indicate that the complement is being used and that the disease is active. So serum complement levels are used, not for diagnosis, but for following the progress of the disease and the response to therapy.[43, 44]

In routine laboratory tests, the patient usually has an elevated sedimentation rate and an anemia and, in 20 percent of the cases, a false positive serology. The urinalysis is important in that proteinuria and/or hematuria may indicate renal involvement. It is possible to have renal involvement with normal urinary sediment. Therefore, in suspect cases more sophisticated renal function tests such as the creatinine clearance are indicated.

A patient may have proven lupus and yet have negative L.E. cell preps, negative fluorescent ANA antibody tests and negative anti-DNA tests. The diagnosis of SLE is made when a high degree of suspicion is maintained in the presence of multisystem disease or any rheumatic manifestation. If one adds a strongly positive fluorescent antinuclear antibody (FANA) test and an antinative DNA test to the 14 criteria of the American Rheumatism Association, a good set of guidelines becomes available.[45]

Tissue biopsy, of course, can make the diagnosis occasionally when all other tests are negative. Immunofluorescent studies of skin biopsies by competent pathologists are of diagnostic help. A kidney biopsy should not be done routinely. Although it has been noted that there can be renal disease in SLE with normal renal function, if the diagnosis is certain, the kidney biopsy probably would not alter the therapy and subjects the patient to risk. A kidney biopsy is indicated where there is evidence of renal disease, where the diagnosis is in question, and where a positive biopsy would alter the course of therapy. A biopsy is never justifiable for research purposes alone.

Because we are dealing in SLE primarily with women in the childbearing period, the issue of pregnancy frequently arises. In general, there is an increased incidence of spontaneous abortion in patients with the disease; however, many patients have carried successfully to term.[46] Whether or not pregnancy alters the subsequent course of the disease is uncertain.

Another frequent issue is one of the use of contraceptives in the female. Most authorities empirically recommend methods of contraception other than the pill. However, I am inclined to follow Dubois' advice,[40] and although I too recommend that other methods of contraception are preferable, I do not make an issue of it if the patient, recognizing the problem, chooses to continue with the pill.

ON THE TREATMENT OF
SYSTEMIC LUPUS ERYTHEMATOSUS

Considerable talent has been spent in elucidating the etiology and mechanisms involved in systemic lupus erythematosus, yet treatment remains empiric and anecdotal.[47-54]

I tend to base my opinions largely on the work of Dubois, Fries, Holman, and Rothfield, as these are investigators with considerable clinical experience.

Before beginning any therapy or suggesting the diagnosis to the patient, the diagnosis should be firmly established, because it implies a lifetime of disability and possible fatality.

It is important to explain to the patient that he does not have a necessarily fatal disease. In fact, the long-term survival rate is now over 90 percent, and, in cases where there is no renal or central nervous system involvement, the long-term survival rate is excellent. In addition, many cases will have a spontaneous remission.

Before starting therapy, carefully review all medications that the patient is taking to ensure that he does not have a drug-induced disease. Carefully review all physical findings, particularly for signs of infection in the urine or the lungs.

The treatment must be individualized. In the mild, asymptomatic case with minimal findings, reassurance may be sufficient.

If the disease is limited to the discoid type with only a few skin lesions, treatment can consist of local applications of corticosteroid creams and the use of sun screens. The physician should be alert to the fact that long-term use of fluorinated corticosteroid creams may itself produce skin atrophy.

Sun exposure may aggravate the disease in some patients. The patient should be advised to avoid sun exposure and should be instructed in the use of sun screens. To a large extent the patient can help in determining just how much sun exposure is safe.

Rest is an important part of treatment. The patient is chronically fatigued, and the fatigue is organic. He should be encouraged to heed that sign and to recognize that he does not have the sustained physical ability of many of his friends.

If the program of reassurance, rest, and topical steroidal creams is not adequate, then the patient should be treated with the various nonsteroidal anti-inflammatory drugs. (This refers to all anti-inflammatory drugs; it does not refer to gold.) One should recognize that these patients are usually thought to have drug sensitivities and are more likely to over-react to even the simpler drugs than the ordinary patient. Holman, for example, warns that the salicylates in systemic lupus should not be pushed to their maximum tolerance.

If the anti-inflammatory drugs are not adequate, then antimalarials are added to the program. The use of antimalarials dates back to 1894 when quinine was tried in the treatment of discoid lupus erythematosus. Since then, pamaquine (Primaquine), quinine, quinacrine (Atabrine), chloroquine (Aralen), amodiaquine (Camoquin) and hydroxychloroquine (Plaquenil) all have been tried with varying degrees of success in the treatment of both discoid and systemic lupus erythematosus. Although the antimalarials have never been "double blinded," it is Dubois' opinion that 90 percent of patients with discoid systemic lupus erythematosus and 95 percent of the skin lesions in patients with systemic lupus erythematosus will show marked to moderate benefit if the physician uses the drugs properly. In addition, a high percentage of the patients with arthralgias will improve.

The generally accepted procedure is to start with hydroxychloroquine (Plaquenil) 200 mg twice a day. This is the maximum recommended dosage for an adult weighing over 45 kg or 100 lb (5 mg to 7 mg per kg of hydroxychloroquine per day have been used for the long-term treatment of juvenile rheumatoid arthritis without retinal damage). Nevertheless, eye examinations at regular intervals should not be neglected. Improvement on this program should occur within 30 to 90 days. If it does not occur, there is no point in continuing the drug. If it does occur, then the drug should be continued indefinitely. At the end of one year, a slow decrease in dosage should be attempted. Thus, the patient can be reduced to 300 mg daily for three or four months, then 200 mg daily for three or four months. The withdrawal should be cautious and slow and should be increased to the maintenance dose if there is an exacerbation. Under no circumstances should the maximum recommended dosages be exceeded. If the patient cannot tolerate Plaquenil because of a skin rash or a gastrointestinal disturbance, then chloroquine (Aralen) in a dosage of 250 mg daily may be substituted. This is the maximum adult dosage and assumes a minimum weight of 45 kg or 100 lb (chloroquine in a dose of 4 mg/kg per day has been used in juvenile rheumatoid arthritis without retinal damage).

The chloroquine should be used in the same way that the Plaquenil was used, slowly decreasing the dosage at the end of one year.

If the chloroquine or Plaquenil are not successful, then mepacrine (Atabrine) 100 mg daily may be added to the program. Thus chloroquine is never added to the Plaquenil program, because both chloroquine and Plaquenil are toxic to the retina. Atabrine in the recommended dosage is not toxic to the retina and therefore can be added synergistically to either chloroquine or Plaquenil. No one knows the long-term toxicity of 100 mg of Atabrine daily, but apparently it is a reasonably safe maintenance dose that can be used for years if necessary and if properly monitored aplastic anemia has been reported.

As discussed in the chapter on chloroquine and Plaquenil, the most serious side effect of these two drugs is retinal toxicity and resulting blindness. However, if the recommended dose is not exceeded, the risk appears to be reasonable. It is essential, however, that any patient placed on these drugs have a baseline ophthalmologic examination and then have regular ophthalmologic tests every three to six months.

Atabrine taken for long periods of time may cause a yellow staining of the skin which may suggest jaundice. However, it is not a contraindication to continuing with the drug.

Other side effects, as discussed in the chloroquine chapter, include nausea, vomiting, dermatitis, diarrhea, personality changes, itching, psychosis, convulsive seizures, severe leukopenia, gray hair, myasthenia, cycloplegia, thrombopenia, cramps, and aplastic anemia. For the most part these side effects are rare. The physician, however, should be particularly alert to the development of a myasthenia which is very difficult to distinguish from rheumatoid arthritis. Another side effect recently recognized as a result of chloroquine and Plaquenil is a chronic pigment disturbance of the skin which may appear after long-term therapy.

The antimalarials are of little value during the treatment of acute crisis in systemic lupus, nor do they seem to alter the course of the disease when there is renal involvement. When added to steroid therapy, however, they seem to be particularly effective in permitting a reduction in the dosage of steroids.[55]

There will be very few failures in patients with systemic lupus treated, as previously outlined. In a few cases it may be necessary to add small amounts of steroids. It is suggested that it would be well to start with prednisone 1 mg tablets, using 1 or 2 mg daily every morning and slowly increasing the dose as necessary. Never exceed 7-10 mg daily, except in patients with renal or hematologic or central nervous system involvement.

Most physicians empirically use steroids in acutely ill patients. The dosage is empiric. Dubois recommends the following dosage schedule of prednisone:

Hemolytic anemia: 60-80 mg, increasing to 100-120 mg daily if improvement does not occur within a week.

Thrombocytopenic purpura: 80 mg per day; it may take as long as four weeks to see a result.

Polyserositis: 40-60 mg per day; response should be prompt.

Acute vasculitis: 40-100 mg per day; response should occur in a few days, except for the gangrene of the extremities which may take several weeks to improve.

Acute central nervous system damage: 50-100 mg every 12 hours. If there is no response in 24-48 hours, then change to intravenous glucocorticosteroids such as hydrocortisone sodium succinate, (Solu-Cortef) 50-500 mg intramuscularly or intravenously every 12 hours, and double the dose every 24-48 hours to 3,000 mg daily, then maintain it at that level for several weeks until the patient is cushingoid.

Renal damage: 50-60 mg per day or 100-120 mg every other day. Improvement usually requires 8-12 weeks.

LUPUS STEROID THERAPY

Large doses of steroids used for acute hemolytic anemia, thrombocytopenic purpura, acute vasculitis, acute central nervous system damage, and renal damage usually require at least two or three months of therapy before definite benefit can be observed. After this period of time, the dosage of steroids is slowly reduced. This requires a certain amount of clinical experience. The longer the patient has been on large doses of steroids and the higher the dosage, the more difficult the withdrawal. In patients who have been on large doses for long periods of time, the withdrawal should be extremely slow, and only clinical judgment can determine whether or not the withdrawal is too rapid. If an exacerbation occurs during the withdrawal, the dosage should be increased. As a rule of thumb, 10 percent of the dosage may be reduced at intervals as short as four days or, in more severe cases, the 10 percent reduction may occur at intervals of a few weeks. At the higher levels, the dosage reduction may be rather rapid, but the lower the dosage, the slower the reduction. Some patients may be particularly sensitive to even a small dosage reduction. Thus, a patient on 5 mg of prednisone daily may notice even a 0.5 mg reduction, but this does represent 10 percent of the total dose. As one approaches the lower levels, the use of 1 mg tablets helps in careful titration.

Large-dose steroid therapy produces many problems. Among the worst is psychosis. Sometimes it is difficult to decide whether the psychosis is due to the underlying disease or to the large doses of steroids. It is important to bear in mind that a steroid induced psychosis can be superimposed upon an organic psychosis in these patients and that the drug-induced psychosis may not be recognized until there is total cessation of steroid therapy. Chlorpromazine is a useful agent for managing these psychotic episodes. It does not seem to produce exacerbations of the systemic lupus.

Continued use of large doses of steroids may produce hyperlipoproteinemia, diabetes, abnormal fat distributions, pancreatitis, severe peptic ulcer, pseudotumor cerebri, posterior capsular cataracts, rarely maculopapular or urticarial rashes. There is also evidence that there is an increased incidence of coronary artery disease and myocardial infarction. There is a definite increased incidence of infections in these patients who are more susceptible to herpes zoster, which may be fatal, and to fungal infections. Myopathy is not unusual in long-term steroid therapy and may be difficult to distinguish from the underlying disease. One therefore has to recognize that high-dosage steroid therapy in the treatment of systemic lupus is fraught with complications and demands a certain amount of skill and experience.

THE IMMUNOSUPPRESSIVES

A recent survey indicated that 25 percent of practicing "experts" would use either Cytoxan or azathioprine in the treatment of systemic lupus, especially in the presence of renal involvement. Most would use these drugs in combination with the corticosteroids hoping to lessen the need for large doses of steroids. A few would use these drugs with very little or no steroids. The results of therapy in the New Zealand rat lupus model with immunosuppressives are excellent. The results in humans are questionable.

At this time it would appear wise to consider the use of Cytoxan and azathioprine as experimental and leave their use to the investigators. Don't feel guilty if you do not use immunosuppressives. The argument that the disease is fatal, hence a toxic drug is justified, is not valid. You just might be doing your patient a favor if you do not use immunosuppressives.

THE NEUROPSYCHIATRIC
ABNORMALITIES AND NEUROLOGIC CHANGES
IN SYSTEMIC LUPUS ERYTHEMATOSUS
By Robert Rosenbaum

Clinicians have known for the last 100 years that there is a high incidence, estimated to be from 25-50 percent, of neuropsychiatric abnormalities and organic neurologic disease in patients

with systemic lupus. Occasionally, the neuropsychiatric manifestations or the neurologic manifestations may be the presenting symptom. Because these patients have a chronic disease,
there is adequate exogenous reason for neuropsychiatric manifestations. In addition, many of these patients as a part of their
disease process may have an arteritis involving sections of the
brain; some may have episodes of cerebral edema; and others
may have autoimmune complexes deposited in the brain. Most
are on medications such as chloroquine or prednisone, which
may cause seizures and/or psychosis, and may be on immunosuppressives which make them vulnerable to exotic subclinical
infections. Furthermore, a certain incidence of neurologic and
psychiatric disease exists in any group or population.

When we consider all of these variables, the number of psychiatric manifestations and/or neurologic manifestations that a patient with lupus may exhibit become unlimited. Clinically,
therefore, we read of innumerable bizarre cases that ultimately
are diagnosed as lupus. I myself have had the experience of seeing a few patients treated as schizophrenic for a number of years
until peripheral joint swelling made the diagnosis of systemic
lupus obvious. The psychoses of these patients responded dramatically to chloroquine. Holman reports cases with transverse
myelitis, idiopathic internal hydrocephalus, idiopathic cerebral
edema, and coma. Dubois reports patients with classic symptoms of multiple sclerosis, who, on ultimate examination, were
found to have a multisystem disease, systemic lupus.

The following neurologic signs have all been listed as manifestations of lupus: convulsions, hemaplesia, double vision, choked
discs, polyneuritis, subarachnoid hemorrhage, nystagmus, vertigo, choreiform movement, monoplegia, paraplegia, quadra-
plegia, aphasia, intention tremor, Bell's palsy, cortical blindness, and decerebrate state. In addition to all of these central
nervous findings, peripheral neuritis of varying degrees of severity has been reported in 9-12 percent of systemic lupus patients. Psychoses have been reported in up to 12 percent of the
cases, and may take multiple forms such as schizophrenia, para-
noia, or catatonic states.

There is no single pathognomonic lesion which can account for
all of these manifestations. The pathophysiology may vary from
small vessel arteritis to thrombocytopenia or to a wide variety
of immunologic abnormalities.

Because of the various pathophysiologies and because of the multiple areas of the brain involved, diagnosis is a challenge. The
diagnosis depends first on making a diagnosis of systemic lupus

erythematosus and then developing a high degree of suspicion that the central nervous system symptoms may be part of the basic disease. One must be careful, however, because these patients, just as those in the general population, are subject to infectious encephalitis, neoplasms, brain tumors, and subdural hematomas. A wide variety of abnormalities have been reported in the neuropsychiatric signs and symptoms of lupus. The problem is that these findings are never consistent. Thus, although cells may be present in the spinal fluid, they may be absent when the lesion is deep. The EEG may be either abnormal or normal.

There is no uniformity of therapy in the treatment of neurologic aspects of the disease.

All authorities agree that anticonvulsants are indicated in the treatment of the seizure disorders. Dubois in 1974 felt that the antimalarials should be discontinued in patients developing psychoses and seizures. This is contrary to my personal experience. Many physicians use prednisone; others believe it to be of no value because it may cause psychosis.

As for treatment, I prefer to generally follow the recommendations of Fries and Holman. (1) Central nervous system disease is not necessarily an ominous finding. Survival from an acute episode is not necessarily followed by a second occurrence. There are multiple causes for the neurologic syndromes, and treatment of the basic disease is of primary importance. (2) A patient with neurological involvement should have general supportive care, including monitoring and control of blood pressure, use of platelet transfusion when indicated, and the early employment of antibiotics if a specific infection is identified either in the central nervous system, the blood, or the urine. (3) Anticonvulsants are indicated in seizure disorders. (4) Chloroquine is not contraindicated in central nervous system involvement and should be used as in the chapter on chloroquine. (5) Consider the possibility that the patient may be over-reacting to the drugs, particularly prednisone and possibly even the so-called minor anti-inflammatory agents such as aspirin, phenylbutazone, indomethacin, etc.

THE PROBLEMS OF SYSTEMIC LUPUS ERYTHEMATOSUS

Pregnancy is not contraindicated in patients with systemic lupus, but there is a high risk of miscarriages in this population. The problem is further complicated by the fact that systemic lupus does not go into remission with pregancy and may necessitate drug therapy. The effect of drugs on the fetus is always unknown.

THE CONTRACEPTIVE PILLS

Because patients with systemic lupus tend to be particularly drug-sensitive, physicians have usually advised against the use of contraceptive pills. On the other hand, pregnancy is not particularly desirable in these patients. Dubois sums it up best when he relates that he usually advises these patients not to take contraceptive pills, but he is not too disturbed if they ignore his advice.[47]

INFLUENZA VACCINATIONS

In general, because we think of this disease as being an "autoimmune disease," we have tended to advise our patients not to take parenteral injections. Recent studies, however, have demonstrated that influenza vaccinations have produced no harmful effects in this disease, and, because these people do poorly when they develop infectious illnesses, it is probably preferable that they receive influenza vaccinations.

PRINCIPLES OF TREATMENT

1. Do not treat until the diagnosis is established.

2. Do not overtreat. The mild cases can be handled with reassurance, aspirin, and the newer nonsteroidal anti-inflammatory drugs, or indomethacin or phenylbutazone.

3. These patients are particularly susceptible to infection. When an exacerbation occurs, it may not necessarily be due to an exacerbation of the disease. Examine the patient carefully for infections involving the kidneys, the heart, or the lungs.

4. Advise a reasonable period of rest.

5. Avoid excessive exposure to the sun but do not make a fetish of it.

6. Chloroquine, hydroxychloroquine, and Atabrine usually will control the skin manifestation and arthralgias.

7. Prednisone in small doses - less than 10 mg a day - may be added to the program when the patient does not respond to more conservative management.

8. The complications are usually treated aggressively with large doses of steroids until the active manifestation of the disease

subsides. Then the dosage is slowly and gradually reduced over a period of months. The following are some of the conditions in which one would consider large doses of steroids:

a) Early clinical nephritis. It is probably wise to treat this to prevent the progression of the disease.

b) When there is an active nephritis with a rising creatinine, large doses of steroids are indicated.

c) Serologic flare in which there is a rising anti-DNA and a drop in serum complement are treated aggressively by some physicians. There is no unanimity of opinion regarding this. My own personal choice is watchful waiting. I believe in treating the patient, not the laboratory; and I recommend not increasing the doses of steroids but watching to see what develops.

d) Central nervous system involvement demands large doses of steroids.

When large doses of prednisone are used, tapering usually starts when clinical manifestations of the disease subside. As an example, if prednisone was given in a dosage of 60 mg a day, one would hope to be at 33 mg in three months, 17 mg at six months, and under 10 mg by eight or nine months. However, during this period of time, if there was a clinical and laboratory flare-up, one would increase the prednisone.

There are some physicians who would treat these patients with immunosuppressives. However, the majority of rheumatologists do not use immunosuppressives. I think it is best at this time to consider the immunosuppressives as definitely being in the experimental class. Their use should be limited to scientific clinical investigation.

There are no absolutes in the treatment of this disease. Treatment is largely empiric and each patient must be individualized.

SUMMARY

Lupus is a disease in which an antigen antibody reaction plays an essential role.

ANTIGEN   +   ANTIBODY

DNA   IgG

Serum Complement

May involve:

Brain	-	Psychosis - seizures
Heart	-	Pericarditis
Kidneys	-	Nephritis - nephrosis
Skin	-	Rashes
Joints	-	Arthralgias
Blood	-	Hemolytic anemia
		Thrombocytopenia
Lungs	-	Pleural effusion

DIAGNOSES: Consider Lupus

1. Arthralgias and arthritis associated with leukopenia, proteinuria, hematuria, false positive test for syphilis
2. Idiopathic fever
3. Unexplained hemolytic anemia; thrombocytopenia
4. Fever of undetermined origin
5. Idiopathic nephrosis or nephritis
6. Unusual psychosis; idiopathic seizures

LABORATORY AIDS

1. Anemia, elevated sedimentation rate

2. Albuminuria, cellular casts

3. L.E. cell prep (only positive in 60 percent of cases - many false positives) requires an expert's interpretation seldom used nowadays

4. Fluorescent antinuclear antibody test - (FANA) requires equipped laboratory (supersensitive - many false positives)

5. Antinative DNA test - most specific; requires specialized laboratory - DNA not standardized so results vary; valuable in that titer rise or fall may be a clue to success of therapy

6. Serum complement - of no value in diagnosis but a low value indicates activity

7. In renal involvement - urea- creatinine - creatinine clearance

DIAGNOSES

1. A high degree of suspicion
2. Check 14 criteria listed on p. 140
3. Positive laboratory tests

PITFALLS

1. Lupus can be present with normal laboratory tests. Consider renal or skin biopsy if these organs are involved.

2. Drugs can simulate the disease. Be sure patient is not on drugs known to cause lupus-like syndrome. Antinative DNA test is negative.

REFERENCES

1. Talbot, J.H.: Lupus Erythematosus. Dubois, E.L. (ed.), University of Southern California Press, Los Angeles, 1976, p. 1.

2. Osler, W.: On the visceral complications of erythema exudativum multiforme. American Journal of Medical Science 110:629, 1895.

3. Libman, E. and Sacks, A.B.: A hitherto undescribed form of valvular and mural endocarditis. Archives of Internal Medicine 33:701, 1924.

4. Gross, L.: Cardiac lesions in Libman-Sacks disease with consideration of its relationship to acute diffuse lupus erythematosus. American Journal of Pathology 16:375, 1940.

5. Baer, G., et al.: A diffuse disease of the peripheral circulation usually associated with lupus erythematosus and endocarditis. Transactions of the Association of American Physicians 50:139, 1935.

6. O'Leary, P.A.: Prognosis and treatment of lupus erythematosus. Mayo Clinic Proceedings 16:686, 1940.

7. Hargraves, M.M., et al.: Presentation of two bone marrow elements: The "tart" cell and the L.E. cell. Mayo Clinic Proceedings 23:25, 1948.

8. Hargraves, M.M.: L.E. cell phenomenon. Mayo Clinic Proceedings 27:419, 1952.

9. Hargraves, M.M.: Production in vitro of the L.E. cell
    phenomenon: Use of normal bone marrow elements and
    plasma from patients with acute disseminated lupus erythe-
    matosus. Mayo Clinic Proceedings 24:234, 1949.

10. Hargraves, M.M.: Discovery of the L.E. cell and its mor-
    phology. Mayo Clinic Proceedings 44:579, 1969.

11. Beerman, J.H.: The L.E. cell and phenomenon in lupus
    erythematosus. American Journal of Medical Sciences 222:
    473, 1951.

12. Dubois, E.L.: Current status of the L.E. cell test. Semi-
    nars in Arthritis and Rheumatism 1:97, 1971.

13. Monto, R.W., et al.: The L.E. cell: Significance and Re-
    lationship to Collagen Disease - Inflammation and Diseases
    of Connective Tissue: A Haheman Symposium, Mills, L.C.,
    Moyer, J.H. (eds), W.B. Saunders Co., Philadelphia, 1961.

14. Miescher, et al.: Lupus Erythematosus. Dubois, E.L.,
    (ed.), University of Southern California Press, Los Ange-
    les, 1976, p. 153.

15. Haserick, J.R., et al.: Blood factors in acute dissemi-
    nated lupus erythematosus. American Journal of Medical
    Sciences 219:660, 1950.

16. Blondin, C., et al.: Roles of IgG and IgM antibodies in the
    formation of L.E. cells. Arthritis and Rheumatism 11:94,
    1968.

17. Holman, H., et al.: The reaction of the lupus erythemato-
    sus (L.E) cell factor with deoxyribonucleoprotein of the
    cell nucleus. Journal of Clinical Investigation 38:2059,
    1959.

18. Beck, S.J.: Antinuclear antibodies: Methods of detection
    and significance. Mayo Clinic Proceedings 44:600, 1969.

19. Beck, J.S.: Variations in the morphological patterns of
    "autoimmune" nuclear fluorescence. Lancet 1:1203, 1961.

20. Pincus, T., et al.: Measurement of serum DNA-binding
    activity in systemic lupus erythematosus. The New England
    Journal of Medicine 281:701, 1969.

21. Elling, P.: Reaction of antinuclear factors with polymorphonuclear leukocytes: 1. Absorption studies. Acta Pathologica et Microbiologica Scandinavica 68:281, 1966.

22. Tan, E.M., et al.: Anti-tissue antibodies in rheumatic disease. Arthritis and Rheumatism 20:1419, 1977.

23. McDoffie, et al.: Immunological tests in the diagnoses of rheumatic diseases. Bulletin on Rheumatic Diseases 27, 5 & 6:900, 1976-77.

24. Rothfield, N.E.: Systemic lupus erythematosus. In: Rheumatic Diseases. Katz, W.A., (ed.), J.B. Lippincott Co., Philadelphia, 1977, p. 756.

25. Ruddy, S.: Complement, rheumatic diseases and major histocompatability complexes. In: Rheumatic Diseases: Immunogenetics and Rheumatic Disease. W.B. Saunders Co., Philadelphia, 1977, p. 215.

26. Steinberg, A.D., et al.: Lupus in New Zealand mice and dogs. Bulletin on Rheumatic Diseases 28, 4 & 5:940, 1977-78.

27. Siegel, M.: The epidemiology of systemic lupus erythematosus. Seminars in Arthritis and Rheumatism 3:1, 1973.

28. Winchestor, R.J.: New directions for research in systemic lupus. Arthritis and Rheumatism 21(Supplement):1, 1978.

29. Baldwin, et al.: The clinical course of proliferative and membranous forms of lupus nephritis. Annals of Internal Medicine 73:929, 1970.

30. Estes, D.: The natural history of systemic lupus erythematosus. Medicine 50:85, 1971.

31. Aptekar, R.G., et al.: Deforming nonerosive arthritis of the hands in systemic lupus erythematosus. Clinics in Orthopedics 100:120, 1974.

32. Bliefield, C.J., et al.: The hand in systemic lupus erythematosus. Journal of Bone and Joint Surgery 56A:1207, 1974.

33. Russell, A.S., et al.: Deforming arthropathy in systemic lupus. Annals of Rheumatic Disease 33:204, 1974.

34. Cohen, A.S., et al.: Preliminary criteria for the classification of systemic lupus erythematosus. Bulletin on Rheumatic Diseases 21:643, 1971.

35. Gibson, T.P., et al.: Use of American Rheumatism Association preliminary criteria for the classification of systemic lupus erythematosus. Annals of Internal Medicine 77:754, 1972.

36. Cohen, A.S., et al.: Criteria for classification of systemic lupus erythematosus. Arthritis and Rheumatism 15: 540, 1972.

37. Fries, et al.: Testing the "preliminary criteria" for classification of SLE. Annals of Rheumatic Diseases 32:171, 1973.

38. Duston, H.P., et al.: Rheumatic and febrile syndrome during prolonged hydralazine treatment. Journal of the American Medical Association 154:23, 1954.

39. Perry, H.M., et al.: Syndrome simulating collagen disease caused by hydralazine (Apresoline). Journal of the American Medical Association 154:670, 1954.

40. Lee, S.L.: Drug-induced systemic lupus erythematosus: A critical review. Seminars in Arthritis and Rheumatism 5:83, 1975.

41. Blongren, S.E.: Drug-induced lupus erythematosus. Seminars in Hematology 10:345, 1973.

42. Dubois, E.L.: Current status of the L.E. cell test. Seminars in Arthritis and Rheumatism 1:97, 1971.

43. McDuffie, F.C., et al.: Immunologic tests in the diagnosis of rheumatic disease. Bulletin on Rheumatic Diseases 27:900, 906, 1976-77.

44. Sontheimer, R.D., et al.: An immunofluorescence assay for double-stranded DNA antibodies using Crithidia luciliae kinetoplast as a double-stranded DNA substrate. Journal of Laboratory and Clinical Medicine 91:550, 1978.

45. Fries, J.F., et al.: Systemic Lupus Erythematosus: A Clinical Analysis. W.B. Saunders Co., Philadelphia, 1975.

46. Bresnihan, B.: Immunological mechanisms for spontaneous abortion in systemic lupus erythematosus. Lancet 1: 1205, 1977.

47. Dubois, E.L.: Lupus Erythematosus. University of Southern California Press, Los Angeles, 1976.

48. Urman, J.D. and Rothfiels, N.: Corticosteroid therapy in systemic lupus. Journal of the American Medical Association 238:2272, 1977.

49. Hahn, B.H., et al.: Azathioprine plus prednisone compared with prednisone alone in treatment of systemic lupus. Annals of Internal Medicine 83:597, 1975.

50. Decker, J.L., et al.: Cyclophosphamide or azathioprine in lupus glomerulonephritis. A controlled trial: Results of 28 months. Annals of Internal Medicine 83:806, 1975.

51. Rothfield, N.F.: Immunosuppressive therapy in lupus erythematosus. Annals of Internal Medicine 83:727, 1975.

52. Fries, J.F. et al.: Cyclophosphamide therapy in systemic lupus erythematosus and polymyositis. Arthritis and Rheumatism 16:154, 1973.

53. Kaplan, D.: Treatment of systemic lupus erythematosus. Arthritis and Rheumatism 20 (Supplement):175, 1977.

54. Wasner, C. and Fries, J.F.: Treatment decisions in systemic lupus erythematosus. Arthritis and Rheumatism 21: 601, 1978.

55. Dubois, E.L.: Antimalarials in management of discoid and systemic lupus. Seminars in Arthritis and Rheumatism 8: 33, 1978.

CHAPTER 6:   MIXED CONNECTIVE TISSUE DISEASE

Rheumatologists have long recognized that the symptoms of some patients defy categorization. These patients appear to suffer from systemic lupus, scleroderma, rheumatoid arthritis, and polymyositis. In 1971, Sharp demonstrated that some of these patients had a specific serologic characteristic; their sera agglutinated a specific antibody, nuclear ribonucleoprotein (RNP) in unusually high titers.[1,2]

Most of these people present with arthralgias and frank joint swelling. Often their hands look like those of patients with rheumatoid arthritis, which is frequently the initial diagnosis.[3] It is the atypical clinical pattern that usually alerts the clinician to the proper diagnosis. The hands may have a diffuse swelling leading to tapered or sausage-like appearance of the fingers; Raynaud's phenomenon occurs, as does esophageal hypomotility and inflammatory myositis. Some of these patients also exhibit pulmonary disease, lymphadenopathies, skin rashes, diffuse sclerodermal changes, serositis, splenomegaly and hepatomegaly.[4] Patients rarely have renal involvement, but this can occur.[5]

Laboratory abnormalities that often occur in mixed connective tissue disease are an elevated sedimentation rate, moderate anemia, leukopenia, a Coombs' positive hemolytic anemia, thrombocytopenia, elevated muscle enzymes in the serum, and diffuse hypergammaglobulinemia. The important distinguishing serologic feature is that almost all patients with mixed connective tissue disease have high titers, usually 1:1,000 to 1:10,000,000 of an agglutinating antibody to a nuclear antigen extracted from isolated nuclei and termed extractable nuclear antigen (ENA). Sharp's contribution was demonstrating that if an extract was prepared of isolated cell nuclei, the sera would agglutinate an unknown antigen in this extract in high titers, thus, hopefully distinguishing these patients from patients with systemic lupus erythematosus. However, it was soon appreciated that sera of patients with SLE would also agglutinate extractable nuclear antigen (ENA). Sharp and others then proceeded to further purify this antigen and identify it as nuclear ribonucleoprotein (RNP).

The sera of patients with mixed connective tissue disease usually agglutinate this antigen in high titer, while the sera from patients with systemic lupus usually do not.[4]

Patients with mixed connective tissue disease, which appears very responsive to small doses of prednisone, are said to have a reasonably good prognosis.

It is easy to diagnose a patient with mixed connective tissue disease as having rheumatoid arthritis: the patient's hands may appear rheumatoid, with erosive changes on x-ray; a high rheumatoid factor may exist in the serum; the sedimentation rate is frequently elevated, and anemia is often present. Clinically, however, one should be alerted by Raynaud's disease in these patients, swollen hands, esophageal hypomotility and myositis, and sclerodermal changes.

SUMMARY

In patients who exhibit signs of multiple types of inflammatory arthritis with symptoms suggesting rheumatoid arthritis, systemic lupus, scleroderma, and polymyositis, suspect mixed connective tissue disease. The important, almost specific, laboratory finding is the high titer for RNP antigen. The patients have a good life expectancy and respond to small doses of steroids.

REFERENCES

1. Sharp, G.C., et al.: Association of autoantibodies to different nuclear antigens with clinical patterns of rheumatic disease and responsiveness to therapy. Journal of Clinical Investigation 50:350, 1971.

2. Sharp, G.C., et al.: Mixed connective tissue disease: An apparently distinct rheumatic disease syndrome associated with specific antibody to an extractable nuclear antigen (ENA). American Journal of Medicine 52:148, 1972.

3. Halla, J.T. and Hardin, J.G.: Clinical features of the arthritis of mixed connective tissue disease. Arthritis and Rheumatism 21:497, 1978.

4. Sharp, G.C.: Mixed connective tissue disease overlap syndromes. In: Clinics in Rheumatic Disease. W.B. Saunders Co., Philadelphia, 1975, p. 561.

5. Bennett, R.M. and Spargo, B.H.: Immune complex ne-
    phropathy in mixed connective tissue disease. American
    Journal of Medicine 63:534, 1977.

6. Reichlin, M.: Mixed connective tissue disease. Modern
    Topics in Rheumatology. I: 157 (ed.), Hughes, G.R.V.,
    Year Book Publishers, Chicago, 1976.

CHAPTER 7: SCLERODERMA

Scleroderma is usually thought of as a skin disease characterized by hardening and loss of elasticity of the skin so that the
patient is "hidebound." Not only is the skin of the hands involved
but the skin of the upper arms, face, trunk, and lower extremities may be involved.

In its full-blown form when the skin is tight, the fingers flexed
and ulcerated, the facial expression pinched, the disease is easily recognized. The reward is in recognizing the disease early
for at its inception it may mimic rheumatoid arthritis or systemic lupus erythematosus. The problem is that there is no specific diagnostic test for the disease. Even skin biopsy is of little help in the early phases. Therefore, the diagnosis depends
on clinical experience and acumen.

In 80 percent of the cases Raynaud's phenomenon is an initial
symptom but because Raynaud's phenomenon may be due to a
specific etiology or may foreshadow many other diseases such
as systemic lupus, it cannot be considered a diagnostic point.

Like lupus, scleroderma is a multistage and multisystem disease. The skin is usually the primary organ involved but it is
possible to have other systems involved without any skin manifestations. The following list shows a percentage system involvement in a group of 261 patients at the Columbia Presbyte-
rian Medical Center and it is substantially in agreement with reports from other centers:[1]

System	Percent Involved
Skin	90
Raynaud's phenomenon	78
Gastrointestinal	52
Esophagus	52
Small and large bowel	15
Pulmonary	43
Cardiac	40
Pericardial	11

System	Percent Involved
Renal	35
Anemia	27
Articular	25
Hypertension	21
Muscle	20

In addition to being a multisystem disease, scleroderma is also a multistage disease. First, there are edema and redness of the skin. These produce sausage-like swellings of the fingers that can be easily mistaken for rheumatoid arthritis. Then there are atrophy and tightness of the skin and finally, there is the end stage where the skin is hidebound, ulcerated, scarred. The combination of multiple system involvement and multiple stages has produced a variety of syndromes and has created some terminology that is specific to the disease. Sclerodactyly refers to indurative changes involving the fingers distal to the proximal interphalangeal joint.

Acrosclerosis refers to the disease when it is confined to the distal part of the upper extremities and is symmetrical in distribution. The Crest syndrome refers to the association of calcinosis, Raynaud's phenomenon, sclerodactyly, and telangiectasia.

Morphea refers to a localized area of scleroderma which involves only the skin and subcutaneous tissue and may occur anywhere in the body and in any age group. Linear scleroderma refers to a streak of scleroderma anywhere in the body.

There are no laboratory tests that are specific for scleroderma. Often, at the onset of the disease, all laboratory tests are normal. The following laboratory tests may occur but are nonspecific:

1. Anemia
2. Elevated sedimentation rate
3. Hypergammaglobulinemia
4. Positive test for the RA factor
5. Positive tests for L.E. cells and/or antinuclear antibodies

The committee of the American Rheumatism Association, after ten years of study, has developed the following clinical criteria for early diagnosis. The most important clinical finding was sclerodermal involvement proximal to the metacarpal or metatarsal joints (MCP, MTP). This finding is present in 91 percent of the definite cases of scleroderma.

If this one major criterion of scleroderma were absent, diagnosis could still be established if two of the following four minor criteria were present:

1. Sclerodactyly
2. Digital pitting scars
3. Pulmonary fibrosis
4. Colonic sacculations

Other prominent features of the disease, for example, Raynaud's phenomenon, esophageal dysmotility, and low pulmonary diffusing capacity did not improve discrimination.

The prognosis of the disease is indefinite. If it is purely limited to the skin, in the individual case the prognosis may be good. The disease may linger for years, may not shorten life, and may even have remissions. However, the prognosis for the group is poor, particularly when there is organ involvement, especially if the organ involvement is renal. Therefore, one sees all variations of the disease: the mild form that hardly requires treatment and the severe form with a rapid fulminating course and early death.

There is no known treatment that alters the prognosis. The hope is, however, that if one detects early a specific system involvement, some of the treatment now available or one that develops in the future may help to prevent the irreversible fibrosis. Recent reports indicate that aggressive treatment of renal involvement and associated hypertension may alter the prognosis.

Once the diagnosis is established, a thorough examination of all organ systems is indicated and these systems should be re-evaluated as the disease progresses. Thus it is common to order an esophagram, an upper G.I., small and large bowel studies and esophageal motility studies where available. The chest x-ray is done routinely but by the time pulmonary fibrosis is visible on x-ray, the disease is far advanced. Therefore, where available, more sensitive diagnostic techniques such as diffusion capacity, pulmonary blood volume, and even pulmonary artery catheterization may be indicated. Kidney disease manifests itself by hypertension, proteinuria, azotemia, and oliguria. The kidneys should be monitored as carefully as they are in systemic lupus. Cardiac disease may manifest itself by pericardial effusion, myocarditis, or coronary artery disease or cardiac failure. The muscles may become involved and can best be detected by clinical features and studies of muscle enzymes.

Treatment is purely empiric. It is my impression, however, that one should carefully distinguish pure scleroderma from systemic lupus or mixed connective tissue disease because chloroquine and prednisone seem to be effective when scleroderma accompanies these diseases.

The treatment of scleroderma is purely symptomatic. For the Raynaud's phenomenon, guanethidine (Ismelin), 12.5 mg daily for three weeks, then 25 mg for three weeks, then 37.5 mg thereafter; or alpha-methyldopa (Aldomet) 250 mg twice a day for three weeks, 500 mg twice a day for three weeks, then 750 mg twice a day thereafter; or reserpine 0.25 mg twice a day for three weeks, then 0.25 mg three times a day for three weeks, then 0.50 mg twice a day has been recommended.

All of these drugs have side effects and should be carefully monitored, particularly the reserpine which may produce serious depression. No one has shown that the drugs, by altering the symptom of Raynaud's disease, alter the prognosis.

As a general anti-inflammatory agent, aspirin and/or indomethacin seem to offer symptomatic relief. Low doses of prednisone may help the swelling at the early onset of the disease. At the present time experimentation is going on with large doses of prednisone, 40-60 mg at the early detection of pulmonary involvement. In esophageal dysphagia, antispasmodics may be tried. When there is small bowel and large bowel involvement accompaniment, alternating antibiotics to reduce bacterial flora may be helpful. The following regimen has been suggested: tetracycline, 250 mg four times a day for 10 to 14 days followed by a course of ampicillin and neomycin given at a later date if there is a recurrence of symptoms.

SUMMARY

Scleroderma is a disease involving skin, muscles, lungs, heart, kidneys, gastrointestinal tract. If the skin alone is involved, the prognosis may be good. The prognosis is less optimistic if other organs are involved. The initial symptom is often Raynaud's phenomenon. The major diagnostic physical finding is tight skin proximally - the disease at onset may mimic rheumatoid arthritis, lupus, mixed connective tissue disease. Laboratory tests are of limited value in diagnosis. Biopsy of the skin seldom helps. There is no known treatment that alters prognosis. Treatment is symptomatic - aspirin, indomethacin, chloroquine, prednisone.

REFERENCES

1. LeRoy, E.C.: Scleroderma (systemic sclerosis). In: Modern Topics in Rheumatology. Year Book Medical Publishers, Chicago, 1976, p. 151.

2. Rodan, G.P.: The natural history of progressive systemic sclerosis (diffuse scleroderma). Bulletin on Rheumatic Diseases 13:301-304, 1963.

3. Committee of the American Rheumatism Association. Clinical criteria for early diagnosed systemic sclerosis (SS): Preliminary results of a multicenter study meeting of the American Rheumatism Association. Mesa, A.T., et al., (eds.), American Rheumatism Association, New York, 1978.

CHAPTER 8: HLA-B27 ANTIGEN: AN EXPLANATION

By James Rosenbaum

Susceptibility to a wide range of diseases has recently been shown
to be associated with a set of genes on the sixth human chromosome. These genes are called the major histocompatibility complex (MHC) or human leukocyte antigen (HLA) System. Although
the nomenclature can be extremely complex, the clinician's task
is not exceedingly arduous, because at the present time our understanding of HLA has only limited application for the practitioner. However, the rapid expansion of knowledge of immunogenetics offers the hope that an understanding of the HLA system
may soon clarify the pathogenesis of a vast array of diseases.
A little historical background and an introduction to the terminology seems in order.

In the 1950s, antibodies that agglutinated white blood cells (leukoagglutinins) were recognized in the sera of individuals who had
received multiple transfusions. Similar antibodies were found
in some multiparous females.[1,2] These antibodies affected white
blood cells of some but not all normal individuals. Because the
antigens detected were first found on white blood cells, they were
labeled HLA (human leukocyte antigens). An antiserum against
an HLA determinant plus complement will cause lysis of lymphocytes with the appropriate HLA antigen. Using the technique
called microlympho cytotoxicity assay, cells can be readily
HLA-typed by serologic means.[3]

Two major loci or areas on the sixth human chromosome determine HLA antigens. These loci have been labeled "A" and "B."
Each locus has roughly 20 different possible alleles, that is, alternative forms of the same gene.[4] The wide variety of alleles de-
fines the system as polymorphic. Alleles are assigned numbers
based on the agreement of international histocompatibility con-
gresses. If the assignment is tentative, the number is preceded by
a "w" for workshop. Thus, HLA-B27, a particular antigen determined by the B locus, was initially termed BW27. One of the first
recognitions of the importance of the HLA system came in the field
of transplantation. Survival of a renal transplant, for example,

seems to depend on HLA similarity between a donor and recipient.[5] A four-antigen match would mean that the four HLA antigens of the donor (an A locus antigen and a B locus antigen from each parent) were identical to the antigens of the recipient. A third locus can also be detected by serologic means. Termed the "C" locus, it appears to have fewer possible alleles and, at present, less importance for our understanding of HLA-related disease.

A fourth locus appropriately labeled "D" seems likely to be implicated in most diseases that are related to the HLA system. The D locus was initially demonstrated by the mixed lymphocyte reaction (MLR), the ability of irradiated lymphocytes to stimulate another individual's lymphocytes in vitro.[6] So far, only a small number of D alleles have been recognized, but this reflects how cumbersome the search has been; more alleles are likely to be enumerated eventually. Very recently, the probable products of the D locus have been recognized on lymphocytes and noted as DrW1, DrW2, etc. , with the w again indicating the tentative workshop designation and the R indicating related to D. In studies that have included D locus typing, the strongest disease associations have usually been noted. Multiple sclerosis, for example, is associated slightly with HLA-A3 and HLA-B7, but has a strong association with HLA-DW2.[7]

The rheumatologist is the beneficiary of much or our knowledge of the HLA system. Although B27 is present in only 8 percent of the general population, 90 percent of patients with ankylosing spondylitis are B27+.[7] Reiter's syndrome[8] as well as the reactive arthritis that follows a Yersinia or Salmonella infection[7] has a similar strong association with B27. Psoriatic arthritis has a slight association with B27, but a much stronger relation to B13, Bw17, and Bw38.[7] Rheumatoid arthritis is not significantly associated with an A or B allele but has a strong relationship to Dw4.[9]

The association of B27 with ankylosing spondylitis (AS) is the only association which currently might be employed as a diagnostic tool. In a patient suspected of having AS, a test for B27 should have a 10 percent false negative rate and an 8 percent false positive rate, certainly comparable to the reliability of a rheumatoid factor for rheumatoid arthritis. By requesting only B27 rather than complete HLA typing, the physician greatly reduces the cost to the patient. A word of caution is advised: the figures apply only to Caucasian Americans. Among American blacks, for example, only 4 percent of the population carries B27, and roughly only 60 percent of those with AS are B27 positive.

Despite its limited clinical utility thus far, HLA typing has already broadened the understanding of a number of diseases. Approximately 20 percent of "normal" B27 individuals have been shown to have radiographically demonstrable sacroïlitis, regardless of sex.[10] Thus, ankylosing spondylitis may be more prevalent among females than clinically suspected.

The knowledge of the HLA system and its role in immune responses continues to expand. Understanding this antigenic recognition system should provide insight into the pathogenesis of a broad range of disease states.

<h1 style="text-align:center">REFERENCES</h1>

1. Dausset, J.: Leukoagglutinins. IV: Leukoagglutinins and blood transfusion. Vox Sanguinis 4:190-198, 1954.

2. Payne, R.: Leukocyte agglutinins in human sera. Archives of Internal Medicine 99:587-606, 1957.

3. Terasaki, P.I. and McClelland, J.D.: Microdroplet assay of human serum cytotoxins. Nature 204:998-1000, 1964.

4. Payne, R.: The HLA Complex: Genetics and Implications in the Immune Response in HLA and Disease. Dausset, J. and Svejgaard, A., (eds.), Williams and Wilkens, Baltimore, 1977, pp. 26-31.

5. Opelz, G. and Terasaki, P.I.: Tissue typing in renal transplantation. Contemporary Surgery 5:11-17, 1974.

6. van den Tweel, J.G., et al.: Typing for MLC (LD): F. Lymphocytes, from cousin-marriage offspring as typing cells. Transplantation Proceedings 5:1535-49, 1973.

7. Sasazuki, T., et al.: The association between genes in the major histocompatibility complex and disease susceptibility. Annual Review of Medicine 28:425-52, 1977.

8. Morris, R., et al.: HL-A W27 - A clue to the pathogenesis of Reiter's syndrome. The New England Journal of Medicine 290:554, 1974.

9. Stastny, P.: MLC Determinants Associated with Rheumatoid Arthritis in Histocompatability Testing. Kissmeyer-Nielsen, I. (eds.), Munksgaard, Copenhagen, 1975, pp. 797-804.

10. Colin, A. and Fries, J.: Striking prevalence of ankylosing spondylitis in "healthy" W27 positive males and females. A controlled study. The New England Journal of Medicine 293:835, 1975.

CHAPTER 9:   ANKYLOSING SPONDYLITIS
(Rheumatoid Spondylitis)

"The history is diagnostic. They are
worse with rest, better with activity."

Ankylosing spondylitis (rheumatoid spondylitis) is usually considered a disease of young males. It is characterized by chronic
low back pain associated with prolonged morning stiffness. The
stiffness eventually progresses to chronic back pain with a rigid
spine and, in severe cases, a dorsal flexion of the spine resulting in a humped walk.

After recognition that 85 to 90 percent of the patients with rheumatoid spondylitis are HLA-B27 positive, a high incidence of
HLA-B27 positive individuals with psoriatic arthritis, Reiter's
disease, and ulcerative colitis who develop sacroileitis was
noted. As a result, all of these arthritides are sometimes classified as one disease.

Traditionally, teaching has it that ankylosing spondylitis is 10
times as frequent in males as in females. Using HLA-B27 as
markers, recent studies have indicated that the disease occurs
in equal frequency in both sexes and is much more common than
previously thought. Many cases, particularly in females, are
mild and remain undiagnosed.[3,4]

Although there is a juvenile form of the disease, from a practical point of view the disease should be thought of primarily as a
disease of young males in the 20 to 40 age group. Its clinical
importance is that this group is often employed in industry, in
the military, and suffers frequent back sprains, herniated discs,
and direct back injury. Because rheumatoid spondylitis may be
initially accompanied by normal laboratory tests and negative
x-ray findings, these patients are often suspected to be maling-
erers, or needlessly suffer myelograms and disc surgery.

The diagnosis of rheumatoid spondylitis should be considered in
any young male with chronic back pain. Ninety percent of the
patients start with low back pain; 10 percent may start with cervical pain. The classic patient describes awakening with morning stiffness that takes considerable time to relieve through activity

and heat, and reappears as the day progresses. It may be associated with night pain. It has been estimated that from 40 to 50 percent of the patients with ankylosing spondylitis will have uveitis preceding or accompanying the disease.[5,6] In some patients, peripheral joint involvement, primarily of the hips, knees, or heels, may precede the onset of spinal involvement. A very small percentage of patients have associated evidence of systemic disease - anorexia and weight loss.

The earliest clinical finding in rheumatoid spondylitis is decreased chest expansion due to costovertebral involvement. The normal male should have a chest expansion of at least two inches and the female almost as much. Chest expansion will be markedly decreased in the patient with rheumatoid spondylitis. However, as this finding is somewhat subjective, it should be rechecked. Other early physical signs are definite tenderness over the sacroiliac joint, pain in the sacroiliac joints on pelvic compression, and decrease in motion of the spine. This can be confirmed by having the patient bend forward with the knees straight and seeing if the fingers can touch the floor; having the patient stand with heels and back against the wall and seeing if the occiput can touch the wall without elevating the chin, and by performing the Schober test in which a mark is made at the fifth lumbar vertebra (at the level of the iliac crest) and then another mark is made 10 cm directly above. The patient then bends forward and the distance between the two marks is measured. This distance should exceed 5 cm unless there is early lumbar involvement.

The earliest x-ray changes are in the sacroiliac joints and evidence the advance of the disease. The upper third of the sacroiliac joint is not involved, but initially, due to the inflammatory process going on, the lower third of the sacroiliac joint is hazy or fuzzy in appearance. As the disease progresses, the joint develops erosions and may often give the illusion of being widened due to osteoporosis. These joint x-rays must be specifically ordered; they are not taken as part of a routine x-ray examination of the spine. Other early x-ray changes occur in the lumbar vertebra where, as a result of erosion of the anterior corners, the vertebra loses its scalloped longitudinal appearance and is described as being square. The calcification that occurs in the anterior longitudinal ligaments and the eventual bamboo appearance on x-ray are late manifestations of the disease which should have been previously diagnosed.

Although a mild anemia and a slight elevation of sedimentation rate occur in over 80 percent of the patients, 20 percent of the patients have neither an anemia nor an elevated sedimentation rate early in the disease. This adds to the difficulty of diagnosis.

The introduction of genetic tissue typing and the discovery that 85 to 90 percent of the patients are HLA-B27 positive has given us another peg in the diagnosis. However, it should not be used as the sole criterion, because 8 percent of the normal population is HLA-B27 positive, and 10 to 15 percent of the patients with rheumatoid spondylitis (in some racial groups, this may be even higher) are HLA-B27 negative. The spondylitis in these patients, as far as its clinical course or therapy is concerned, differs in no way from the spondylitis associated with the HLA-B27 positive individual.

There is a high incidence of carditis and aortitis in this disease. Aortitis may manifest itself by an aortic insufficiency first detected as an aortic diastolic murmur. In many cases, before the murmur appears the patient may complain of precordial pain or attacks of tachycardia, or cardiac enlargement may be found on x-ray. A prolonged PR interval greater than 0.24 seconds should arouse suspicion of a carditis.[7]

Statistical studies indicate that ankylosing spondylitis may be life threatening, at least to men, because systemic vascular degeneration is one long-term consequence of the disease.[8]

The treatment of rheumatoid spondylitis should begin with patient education. Most of these patients do have a chronic, progressive, painful disease but, with medical management, are able to carry on successfully in nonphysical occupations. There are exceptions. I have even personally seen patients with rheumatoid spondylitis in military combat.

The most important part of the initial therapy is an educational course by the physiotherapist. The patient should be taught proper gait, proper posture, breathing exercises, and "measuring up" every morning. A mark should be placed on the wall and the patient should measure up to that height every day to be certain that he is not developing dorsiflexion of the spine.

Because of the rigidity and osteoporosis of the spine, minor trauma can cause fractures and dislocations and cord damage may produce various neurologic symptom complexes.[11,12]

Amyloidosis as the result of the chronicity of the disease in long-standing cases should be suspect, particularly in the presence of proteinuria. Rectal biopsy is the easiest way to make a diagnosis.[13]

Pulmonary involvement characterized by fibrosis has also been reported.[14]

Anterior uveitis occurs in 10 to 60 percent of the patients with spondylitis. It may precede the onset of the disease or accompany it. It may be recurrent and it may be bilateral. It may be mild or it may be severe enough to result in glaucoma, cataracts, and anterior and posterior synechiae.

The traditional therapy was x-ray therapy. It was very successful in symptomatically relieving the patient for long periods of time, but was abandoned when demonstrated to cause various forms of later malignancy.[9]

As for specific therapy, aspirin is the drug of choice in the milder cases. Adequate reports on the newer anti-inflammatory agents have still not appeared, but there are suggestions in the literature that naproxen may be effective.[10]

The drug of choice is phenylbutazone, oxyphenbutazone, or indomethacin. The usual dosage schedule for the phenylbutazone or oxyphenylbutazone is 100 mg four times a day after meals and at bedtime with food or milk. After relief is obtained, the drug is reduced to a minimum effective dose, often 100 or 200 mg a day. These drugs are so effective in spondylitis that, in my experience, I would suspect the diagnosis if the patient does not respond.

Indomethacin 25 to 50 mg up to four times a day is the usual starting dose. These drugs are limited by their side effects but in my experience can be continued indefinitely in most patients. The newer nonsteroidal anti-inflammatory agents have been reported to be effective in ankylosing spondylitis. Sulindac is approved for therapy in this disease.

REFERENCES

1. Schlosstein, L., et al.: High association of an HL-A antigen, W-27 with ankylosing spondylitis. The New England Journal of Medicine 288:704, 1973.

2. Moll, J.M.H., et al.: Associations between ankylosing spondylitis, psoriatic arthritis, Reiter's disease, and intestinal arthropathies and Behcet's syndrome. Medicine 53:343, 1974.

3. Calin, A., et al.: Striking prevalance of ankylosing spondylitis in "healthy" W-27 positive males and females. The New England Journal of Medicine 293:835, 1975.

4. Ankylosing spondylitis and its early diagnosis (Editorial). Lancet 2:591, 1977.

5. Lipsky, W.: Anterior uveitis and ankylosing spondylitis (Letter). Journal of the American Medical Association 239:191, 1978.

6. Brewerton, D.A., et al.: Acute anterior uveitis and HLA-B27. Lancet 2:994, 1973.

7. Graham, D.G., et al.: The carditis and aortitis of ankylosing spondylitis. Bulletin on Rheumatic Diseases 9:171, 1958.

8. Radford, E.P., et al.: The New England Journal of Medicine 297:572, 1977.

9. Court Brown, W.M., et al.: Mortality from cancer and other causes after radiotherapy for ankylosing spondylitis. British Medical Journal 2:1327, 1965.

10. Hill, H.F., et al.: Naproxen in ankylosing spondylitis. Scandinavian Journal of Rheumatology (Supplement) 2:121, 1973.

11. Lee, M., et al.: Neurological complications of ankylosing spondylitis (Letter). British Medical Journal 1:798, 1962.

12. Russel, M., et al.: The cauda equina syndrome of ankylosing spondylitis. Annals of Internal Medicine 78:557, 1973.

13. Jayson, M.I., et al.: Amyloidosis in ankylosing spondylitis. Rheumatology Rehabilitation 11:78, 1971.

14. Applerouth, D.: Pulmonary manifestations of ankylosing spondylitis. Journal of Rheumatology 2:446, 1975.

CHAPTER 10:   PSORIATIC ARTHRITIS

> The Cat: And this time it vanished quite
> slowly, beginning with the end of
> the tail, and ending with the grin,
> which remained some time after
> the rest of it had gone . .
> "Well! I've often seen a cat
> without a grin," thought Alice,
> "but a grin without a cat!"
>
> Alice in Wonderland

> The Cheshire Cat syndrome: There may be
> only a bare trace of psoriasis. But that does
> not mean that it has not been there and that it
> won't come back.

Psoriatic arthritis is distinct from rheumatoid arthritis. It has
been long recognized that there is an increased incidence of psoriasis associated with rheumatoid arthritis. Only recently has
it been recognized that there is a specific form of arthritis associated with psoriasis.[1] Although psoriatic arthritis is always
associated with psoriasis, the psoriasis may precede the joint
symptoms by years. At times, the evidence of psoriasis may
be minimal, there being only a few nail lesions or minor lesions
around the hairline or over the elbow. Where the psoriasis is
barely found, I have heard it cleverly referred to as the "Che-
shire cat" syndrome.

Psoriatic arthritis may manifest itself in a number of ways, but
the most common form is asymmetrical and oligoarticular.
There is a tendency for involvement of the peripheral joints which
assume a characteristic "sausage" swelling.[2] In contrast to
rheumatoid arthritis, in psoriatic arthritis there may be involvement of the terminal phalangeal joints. In a few patients,
the arthritis is symmetrical and resembles rheumatoid arthritis; in a small percentage of the cases, joint and bone destruction is so extensive that there is telescoping of the digits. There
is an increased incidence of HLA-B27 positive antigens in psoriatic

176

arthritis, and when present, spondylitis resembling classic rheumatoid spondylitis is a common complication.[3]

The roentgenogram presents distinct features, convincing evidence that this is a disease different from rheumatoid arthritis. First, there is a prédilection for the DIP joints with relative sparing of the metacarpophalangeal and metatarsophalangeal and proximal interphalangeal joints. Second, there is whittling or pointing of the terminal phalanges. Third, in a few cases there may be advanced changes showing marked joint destruction due to osteolysis and ankylosis. Fourth, there is lack of symmetry. Fifth, there is a pencil-in-cup appearance, and sixth, there may be an atypical spondylitis. There appears to be little doubt that there are several radiologic features which appear to be almost specific or characteristic of psoriatic arthritis.[4]

Psoriatic arthritis must be distinguished primarily from rheumatoid arthritis. Its distinguishing features are its peripheral joint involvement, the fact that it is almost always serologically negative, the presence of psoriasis even in minute amounts, and the classic radiologic changes.

Usually the disease carries a good prognosis, particularly when it remains confined to the small joints.[4] However, in exceptional cases, the disease may be progressive and crippling and demand therapy.

Gold therapy is considered to be effective in psoriatic arthritis. At one time, it was felt to be ineffective and to have increased toxicity, but recent studies have proved that in fact it does not have increased toxicity and may be even more effective in psoriatic arthritis than it is in rheumatoid arthritis.[5] The dosage of gold salt in psoriatic arthritis is the same as that in rheumatoid arthritis.

In desperate situations, the immunosuppressive drugs have been tried. Their use is still controversial, but if one is going to be used, methotrexate would appear to be the drug of choice. It has been beneficial for severe psoriasis and has helped a few patients with psoriatic arthritis.[6]

REFERENCES

1. Baker, H.: Epidemiological aspects of psoriasis and arthritis. British Journal of Dermatology 78:249, 1966.

2. Moll, J.M.H., et al.: Psoriatic arthritis. Seminars in Arthritis and Rheumatism 3:55, 1973.

3. McClusky, O.E.: HLA-27 in Reiter's syndrome and pso-riatic arthritis. A genetic factor in disease susceptibility and expression. Journal of Rheumatology 1:263, 1974.

4. Wright, V., et al.: Psoriatic arthritis. Bulletin on Rheu-matic Diseases 21:627, 1971.

5. Dorwart, et al.: Chrysotherapy in psoriatic arthritis. Ar-thritis and Rheumatism 21:513, 1978.

6. Podurgiel, B.J., et al.: Liver injury associated with meth-otrexate therapy for psoriasis. Mayo Clinic Procedures (Notes)48:787, 1973.

CHAPTER 11: ARTHRITIS ASSOCIATED WITH ENTERITIS

"Which comes first - the chicken or the egg?
Be alert, the arthritis can precede the enteritis."

Ten to 20 percent of patients with inflammatory bowel disease, Crohn's disease (terminal ileitis), ulcerative colitis, granulomatous bowel disease, or ulcerative proctitis will have a peripheral polyarthritis and/or a spondylitis. Although the peripheral arthritis does not closely resemble rheumatoid arthritis because it tends to be large joint, asymmetrical, and often nondeforming, it can be mistaken for rheumatoid arthritis. The spondylitis resembles that of a classic rheumatic spondylitis. The RA test is negative in the arthritis that accompanies these enteritises. The incidence of HLA-B27 antigen in patients with enteric bowel disease is the same as that of the general population, but the patient with enteric bowel disease who is HLA-B27 antigen positive is much more prone to develop the ankylosing spondylitis.[1-4] In 10 percent of the patients, the arthritis antedates the onset of bowel symptoms.[5] Spondylitis may antedate the onset of bowel symptoms in 25 percent of patients.[6,7] In Whipple's disease, joint manifestations may precede the diagnosis of Whipple's disease by as long as one to 35 years.[3]

In every patient in whom one makes a diagnosis of rheumatoid arthritis and in which the RA test is negative (seronegative rheumatoid arthritis), one should consider the possibility of an enteric arthritis. If there is any history of gastrointestinal bleeding or diarrhea, a proctoscopic examination and a small bowel study with a roentgenogram should be performed. In my experience, many of these patients are treated for rheumatoid arthritis. After many years, sudden development of diarrhea and bleeding and discovery of a proctitis or ulcerative colitis will explain the atypical course of the disease.

It is important to distinguish this group of arthritics, because treatment of the colitis helps peripheral arthritis. It has been my practice to treat these patients with a low residue diet and courses of sulfasalazine (Azulfidine) as indicated. In more complex cases, the assistance of a gastroenterologist is beneficial.

Where spondylitis accompanies a colitis, treatment of the underlying colitis does not seem to alter the course of the spondylitis.
These patients should be treated as patients with rheumatoid
spondylitis are treated.

Intestinal bypass operations performed for the treatment of severe obesity may lead to the development of acute or subacute
forms of arthritis, tenosynovitis, polymyalgia, and polyarthral-
gia. Usually these symptoms are mild and transient, but on occasion may be severe or chronic. Most of these symptoms develop within a period of two to three years following surgery and
are usually self-limiting with complete resolution. However,
occasionally they may be so severe as to require the use of anti-
inflammatory agents, even at times small doses of steroids.[8-10]
In a few patients, the arthritis following an intestinal bypass operation has been severe enough for the patient to request a re-
vision of their bypass surgery to normal anatomic sequence. In
such cases, the arthritis has resolved and remained in remission.[8] The occurrence of arthritis in bypass operations has led
to speculation as to whether or not there may be a common de-
nominator in bowel malabsorption and bacterial infection account-
ing for the arthritis one sees in Whipple's disease and inflammatory enteritises.[11]

The arthritis of Whipple's disease does respond to antibiotic
therapy. I am not aware, however, of any reports describing
antibiotic therapy in bypass operations.[12]

REFERENCES

1. Palumbo, P.J., et al.: Musculoskeletal manifestations of
    inflammatory bowel disease. Ulcerative and granulomatous
    colitis and ulcerative proctitis. Mayo Clinic Proceedings
    48:411, 1973.

2. Wilske, K.R. and Decker, J.L.: The articular manifesta-
    tions of intestinal disease. Bulletin on Rheumatic Diseases
    15:362, 1965.

3. LeVine, M.E. and Dobbins, W.D.: Joint changes in Whip-
    ple's disease. Seminars in Arthritis and Rheumatism 3:79,
    1973.

4. Waters, E.G.L. and Ansell, B.M.: Arthritis associated
    with ulcerative colitis. A clinical and pathological study.
    Annals of Rheumatic Disease 17:169, 1958.

5. McQuen, C.: Arthritis accompanying ulcerative colitis. Clinical Orthopedics 59:9, 1968.

6. Fernandez-Herlihy, L.: The articular manifestations of chronic ulcerative colitis. The New England Journal of Medicine 261:259, 1959.

7. Wright, V. and Watkinson, G.: The arthritis of ulcerative colitis. British Medical Journal 2:670, 1965.

8. Duncan, J.: Arthropathy and the intestinal bypass operation for obesity. Journal of Rheumatology 4:15, 1977.

9. Rose, E., et al.: Intestinal bypass operation associated with circulating immune complexes and HLA-B27. Journal of Rheumatism 4:129, 1977.

10. Fernandez-Herlihy, L.: Arthritis after jejunostomy for intractable obesity. Journal of Rheumatology 4(2):135, 1977.

11. Cave, D.R., et al.: Evidence of an agent transmissible from ulcerative colitis tissue. Lancet 1:1311, 1976.

12. Mickelsen, W.M., et al.: Twenty-second rheumatism review. Arthritis and Rheumatism 19:1017, 1976.

CHAPTER 12:   REITER'S SYNDROME

"Used to be an exclusive male province; now some
say women should join. Will they make it?"

In 1916 a young German army lieutenant, Hans Reiter, described
a case of arthritis, conjunctivitis, and urethritis in a young sol-
dier. Although the syndrome had been described at least a hundred years before, Reiter's name became associated with the
disease.[1] For years, the diagnosis was limited to the classic
case of a young male who developed a nongonococcal urethritis
associated with a conjunctivitis and an arthritis a few days after
sexual intercourse. It is now recognized that there are many
variations of the original theme, marked by two distinct types:
one type occurs after sexually transmitted infection of the urethral tract; the other type occurs after an epidemic of diarrhea
with no history of sexual contact. Several epidemics of dysentery have been observed to precede the occurrence of an unusual
number of patients with Reiter's disease.[2]

There have been various attempts to establish an infectious agent
as the etiology of the disease. However, although numerous organisms have been isolated from the urethra, none has specifically been proven to cause the classic syndrome.[3] The patient
with Reiter's disease may present with more than Reiter's original triad. Additional features may include inflammation around
the head of the penis, described as a circinate balanitis; mucosal
ulcerations; pustular lesions of the soles of the feet and occasionally of the hands, described as keratodermia blennorrhagica.
Because some of these features, such as the urethritis or conjunctivitis, may be subclinical, it is customary to tentatively diagnose Reiter's disease if the skin or penile manifestations are
classic in appearance. Unlike rheumatoid arthritis, which is bilateral, the arthritis in Reiter's syndrome is usually acute,
asymmetrical polyarthritis. In addition, sacroileitis, often unilateral, is common. Sausage-shaped fingers may evidence involvement of the hands. Painful heels and involvement of the
Achilles tendon are not unusual. Recent reports that 63 to 96
percent of the patients with Reiter's disease are HLA-B27 positive, as compared to 4 to 8 percent in normal control subjects,

has led to a broadening of the diagnosis.[5,6] The literature contains descriptions of incomplete Reiter's syndrome in young men who present with an atypical arthritis without urethritis or conjunctivitis but with other stigma of the disease, such as heel pain, sausage digits, or sacroileitis.

The diagnosis is based on clinical findings. No specific laboratory tests are known. A mild leukocytosis may be present, the sedimentation rate may be elevated, and synovial fluid examination may show an elevated white count ranging from 5,000 to 20,000 with up to 30 percent polys. However, a much higher white count, suggesting an infectious arthritis, may be present. The differentiation of Reiter's syndrome from gonococcal arthritis is particularly difficult. However, the mucocutaneous manifestations and the keratodermia blennorrhagica involving the soles and the hands are quite specific for Reiter's disease as compared to a gonorrheal arthritis. Of course, a positive joint culture firmly establishes the diagnosis of gonorrhea. Occasionally, the skin lesions may simulate pustular psoriasis, but the presence of oral lesions, conjunctivitis, and genitourinary symptoms separates the Reiter's from the psoriatic arthritis.[1] There is no specific treatment for the disease. Aspirin, phenylbutazone, and indomethacin usually provide prompt relief of symptoms. Tetracycline, 2 gms daily, has no effect on the arthritis but will relieve the urethritis.[1,6] The penile and skin lesions respond to daily bathing and topical applications of corticosteroid ointments. The heel spurs are treated with heel pads in the shoes and occasionally with local injections of corticosteroids.

It has long been taught that Reiter's syndrome is a self-limited disease of short duration. However, recent studies indicate that Reiter's syndrome may be a major chronic rheumatic disease resulting in long-term disability.[7]

SUMMARY

Reiter's disease is primarily a disease of young males, two-thirds of whom are HLA-B27 positive. There are two distinct patterns. One group of patients will develop the disease after sexual intercourse and will have the classic urethritis conjunctivitis and arthritis triad. Another group may develop it without sexual exposure but following an epidemic of dysentery. Complicating factors experienced by patients frequently include an inflammation of the head of the penis, typical pustular lesions involving the soles of the feet and the hands, ulcerations of the mucosa of the mouth, painful heels and Achilles tendons, and unilateral sacroileitis. Because the urethritis, conjunctivitis, and diarrhea may at times be so mild as to be missed, it is now becoming customary to seriously consider a diagnosis of Reiter's disease in a young male, particularly if he is HLA-B27 positive and presents with an asymmetrical polyarthritis of the lower extremities associated with such symptoms as painful heels, sacroileitis or balanitis, or skin rash. The treatment is symptomatic. Recent studies indicate that the prognosis should be guarded, because many afflicted people develop chronic arthritis.

REFERENCES

1. Ford, D.K.: Reiter's syndrome. Bulletin on Rheumatic Diseases 20:588, 1970.

2. Paronen, I.: Reiter's disease: A study of 344 cases observed in Finland. Acta Medica Scandinavica 131:1, 1948.

3. Lassus, A. and Karvonen, J.: Reactive arthritis, Reiter's disease and psoriatic arthritis. In: Clinics in Rheumatic Disease. W.B. Saunders Co., Philadelphia, 1977, p. 281.

4. Brewerton, D.A., et al.: Reiter's disease and HLA-B27. Lancet 2:996, 1973.

5. Arnett, F.C., et al.: Incomplete Reiter's syndrome: Discriminating features and HLA-W27 in diagnoses. Annals of Internal Medicine 84:8, 1976.

6. Catterall, R.D.: Treatment of Reiter's syndrome. Practitioner 207:76, 1971.

7. Callin, A., et al.: The natural history of Reiter's syndrome (RS) in academic and community circles. Arthritis and Rheumatism 21:548, 1978.

CHAPTER 13: INFECTIOUS ARTHRITIS

"Any organism that penetrates the body defenses
can attack and rapidly destroy a joint."

Any pathogen that affects humans can involve a joint. There is
usually a primary focus with the joint secondarily involved but
occasionally the joint is the primary site following trauma or a
joint injection. Whenever arthritis follows chills and fever, a
septic arthritis should be suspected. In the elderly, the immunosuppressed, the alcoholic, the patient with an artificial joint,
and the rheumatoid patient, the systemic manifestations of an
infection may be minimal. In these cases only a high degree of
suspicion results in diagnoses.

The diagnosis is suggested by finding a primary focus such as
a skin pustule, an abscessed tonsil, a pulmonary lesion, a urethritis, a proctitis, or a pelvic lesion and confirmed by the examination of joint fluid with the demonstration of a positive
smear or a positive culture.

Staphylococcus aureus, Streptococcus pyogenes, Streptococcus
pneumoniae, Hemophilus influenzae, Neisseria gonorrhoeae,
Enterobacteriacae, and Pseudomonas sp. are the usual bacterial invaders[1] but any organism can involve a joint, and in fulminating or unusual cases tuberculosis or fungus infection should
be considered.

The joint fluid examination is the crucial diagnostic test. It is
prudent to discuss the problem with the pathologist before pro-
ceeding because some organisms such as the gonococci are demanding in their cultural requirements. Under sterile conditions, with a No. 18 needle, the joint fluid is aspirated and immediately transported to the laboratory, for cooling may destroy
some organisms and a prolonged stay will permit leukocytic destruction of the joint fluid glucose, giving a false glucose reading.[2] On aspiration, the joint fluid should be examined, because
infected joint fluid is unusually purulent in appearance and in the
presence of certain anaerobes may produce a characteristic
odor. Some of the joint fluid should be placed in a test tube with

a small amount of heparin or EDTA to prevent clotting and to facilitate the cell count. The laboratory should be instructed to do a white blood count and differential count, a joint fluid sugar, and appropriate culture and sensitivity tests. At the time that the joint fluid is drawn, a sample of blood should be drawn for blood sugar.

The laboratory should also do Gram's stains, acid fast stains, and a wet mount for fungus. In addition, the joint fluid should be examined under a polarized light microscope for crystals. In infectious arthritis, the joint fluid white blood count ranges from 10,000 to over 100,000 with 90 percent of the cells being polys. Usually, the count is over 50,000. However, early in an infection or in cases that have been already partially treated with antibiotics, the white count may be low. In addition to aspirating and culturing the joint fluid, blood cultures should be drawn and cultures should be taken when indicated from open skin lesions, the throat, the urine, the urethra, the cervix, and the rectum, particularly if gonorrhea is suspected.

If the difference between the sugar content of the blood and the sugar content of the synovial fluid is at least 50 mg percent, an infectious arthritis should be suspected, but a difference of blood sugar alone is not diagnostic.[3-5]

A negative smear or culture does not rule out infectious arthritis. It has been estimated that joint fluid cultures may be positive in only 25 to 50 percent of the cases of gonorrheal arthritis. Therefore, in suspicious cases, multiple joint aspirations for culture and smear are justified.[6]

Some hospitals now use newer techniques for earlier detection of microbial agents. These techniques involve the use of gas chromatography to detect metabolites of micrometabolism or a technique called counter-immunoelectrophoresis. This technique detects bacterial antigens and antibodies.[6,7]

In the adult the gonococcus is the most common cause of pyarthrosis today and presents special problems. Seventy-five percent of the patients will have prodromal symptoms of fever, shaking chills, skin rash, and migratory polyarthritis and tenosynovitis instead of a frank joint effusion. The other 25 percent develop a frankly hot, swollen joint without any prodromal symptoms. In the prodromal stage, blood cultures are usually positive and joint fluid cultures are negative whereas in the monoarticular stage, joint fluid cultures are positive. When gonorrhea is suspected, it is essential that in addition to joint fluid cultures, blood cultures, throat cultures, and rectal cultures, urethral and cervical cultures are obtained.[8]

After the joint fluid is obtained, if there is reasonable evidence that an infectious arthritis exists, antibiotic therapy should be started promptly because delay may mean irreversible joint destruction. The antibiotic of choice can be determined only by culture and sensitivity studies. Before these are available, the best that can be done is an educated guess. Unless the treating physician had had experience, it is wise at this stage to involve either the hospital pathologist or an infectious disease specialist. The educated guess is based on the results of the smear, the age of the patient, and the initial source of infection if known. Thus all gram-negative diplococci are assumed to be gonococci and the initial treatment is penicillin, or tetracycline if the patient is allergic to penicillin. Because of the increasing incidence of penicillinase-resistant Staphylococcus aureus,[10] all gram-positive cocci are first treated with a semisynthetic penicillinase-resistant penicillin such as nafcillin or oxacillin.[4,11] A cephalosporin is an acceptable alternative in a patient who is penicillin allergic. If the smear is a gram-negative bacillus, in children up to two years of age, suspect H. influenzae and treat with ampicillin.[11] Since increasing numbers of H. influenzae are found to be ampicillin-resistant, chloramphenicol may be required. Gram-negative bacilli for all other age groups are usually considered to be entero-bacteriaceae and are treated with an amino glucoside such as gentamicin. Some authors recommend adding carbenicillin to the amino glucoside if a gram-negative organism is seen on Gram's stain.

If no organism is seen in the smear, the first decision is whether to wait and repeat the smear or culture. In uncertain cases, it is wise to repeat the smear and culture two or three times even at intervals as short as six or twelve hours apart. If the decision is made to treat in spite of the fact that no organism is seen on the smear, then the antibiotic of choice is based primarily on the patient's age. Most adults during the years of sexual activity are usually considered to have gonorrheal arthritis and are treated with penicillin. Oral treatment with ampicillin or tetracycline is an acceptable alternative. The infant from six months to two years is treated with ampicillin. The newborn up to six months of age or the adult over 40 are treated with nafcillin, and gentamicin is added to the regimen in the immunosuppressed, debilitated, or toxic patient.[4]

The antibiotic chosen should be given at maximum safe dose intravenously in bolus injections to achieve transient high therapeutic levels of antibiotics. A continuous intravenous drip is

started and the antibiotic is given in divided doses every four to
eight hours "piggyback" to run in over 30 to 60 minutes. Recommended doses are as follows: nafcillin - 20 mg/kg every four
to six hours intravenously; cephalothin must be given intramuscularly or intravenously. One gram intramuscularly every four
hours or 40 mg/kg intravenously every six hours are acceptable
doses. Penicillin G can also be given intramuscularly or intravenously. The suggested starting dose is 50,000 units per kg
intravenously every six hours. In severe infections, doses up
to 100 million units per day intravenously have been given. Tetracycline is used primarily for gonorrheal arthritis. If the patient can take it, it can be given orally - 250 to 500 mg every
six hours for 14 to 21 days. If the patient cannot tolerate it orally, it can be given intravenously using 7.5 mg/kg every six
hours. The suggested dose of ampicillin is 50 mg/kg every six
hours intravenously; gentamicin - 1 to 1.7 mg/kg every eight
hours intravenously. The dose of gentamicin must be carefully
adjusted for renal insufficiency because of nephro- and ototox-
icity. Serum levels should be followed in all patients.[12]

In order to improve antibiotic penetration into the joints, joint
drainage and irrigation with sterile normal saline is required
as often as the joint becomes distended. It may be necessary to
aspirate and irrigate a joint more than once; obtaining the joint
fluid during therapy permits analysis and direct assay for antibiotic concentration. The concentration of the antibiotic in the
joint fluid should be bacteriocidal in a dilution of at least 1:
10.[4]

The duration of therapy depends on clinical judgment. In some
series, gonococcal arthritis has been treated adequately in as
little as three days while tuberculosis has required at least 18
months. Most acute septic arthritides require two to three
weeks of therapy. The intravenous therapy is changed to oral
therapy when the infection appears to be well controlled and the
patient is not toxic.[4]

During the acute phase of the infection, the joint is immobilized
for relif of pain but as soon as the pain lessens and permits it,
passive range of motion should be carried out by the physiotherapist. Throughout the acute phase physiotherapy should be increased as tolerated to prevent ankylosis and permanent loss of
function. In joints that are deep and cannot be effectively aspirated and irrigated, surgical drainage is indicated.[14] The current standard regimen for gonococcal arthritis is 10 million units
of penicillin G divided into four or six doses per day until improvement occurs. This is followed by 2 grams orally of ampicillin to give a total of 10 days of treatment. However, there

are many modifications of this schedule. Shorter courses have been successful and in cases where the patient is allergic to penicillin, tetracycline is used.[15] If a patient with proven gonorrheal arthritis does not respond dramatically and promptly to penicillin, one should suspect a penicillin-resistant gonococcus.[16]

Failure of the patient to respond to antibiotic therapy should lead to a reevaluation of the problem. First, the diagnosis of infectious arthritis should be questioned. Rheumatic fever, Reiter's disease, and gouty arthritis may all simulate an acute infectious arthritis. Rheumatoid arthritis seldom is accompanied by fever.

Rheumatic fever is now a relatively rare disease. It is a disease primarily of young people and can be distinguished by rising antistreptolysin titers, the development of carditis, the excellent response to a full therapeutic dose of aspirin, and the absence of joint destruction.

It is sometimes almost impossible to distinguish Reiter's disease in its initial onset from gonococcal arthritis. The important distinguishing features are the negative cultures, the absence of tenosynovitis and the characteristic dermatologic changes of Reiter's disease as compared to the dermatologic changes of gonorrheal arthritis. The failure to respond to appropriate antibiotic therapy and the chronicity of the course will eventually separate the two diseases. Acute gouty arthritis can occasionally cause a high joint fluid white count and the joint itself may appear to have an associated cellulitis. The diagnosis is made by the history of recurrent monoarticular attacks of arthritis with remission, the finding of uric acid crystals in the joint fluid aspirate and the response to colchicine.

If the diagnosis of infectious arthritis is firmly established and the patient is not responding, one should consider the possibility of an unusual organism, an antibiotic-resistant organism, or inadequate antibiotic dosage. In a case that is not responding, the orthopedist should be consulted about open joint drainage and the procurement of joint parts for direct smears and cultures.

Of course, rare and exotic organisms, including fungi and mycobacteria, may at times cause infectious arthritis and these will require specific antibiotic therapy.

Total joint replacement also has increased the incidence of septic arthritis. One-half to one percent of patients undergoing total hip replacement will develop postoperative deep wound infections[17] and 0.3 percent will develop delayed blood-borne infection late in the prosthetic joint.[18]

Salvage of an infected artificial joint requires close teamwork among the orthopedist, rheumatologist, and infectious disease specialist. Even after a prolonged vigorous battle, the success rate is not high.[19]

X-rays in the diagnosis of infectious arthritis are indicated and are helpful. The initial x-rays may simply show soft tissue and joint swelling, but serial x-rays taken only weeks apart may show rapid joint destruction which would indicate that an infectious process is going on. Radioisotope techniques are also now being introduced to detect inflammatory processes, particularly in the deeper joints. These at this time still must be interpreted with reservation because of frequent false positives.

SUMMARY

1. Suspect an infectious arthritis when arthritis follows chills and fever. Be alert to the possibility of an infectious arthritis even when systemic symptoms are minimal in the elderly, the alcoholic, the patient with rheumatoid arthritis, and the addict.

2. When infectious arthritis is suspected, look for a primary source.

3. The diagnosis is established by joint fluid aspiration and culture:

    a) Use a No. 18 needle to withdraw joint fluid.
    b) Place part of the joint fluid sample in a heparinized tube to facilitate cell count.
    c) Order:
       (1) Gram's stain
       (2) Hanging drop examination
       (3) Culture
       (4) White blood count and differential, blood sugar
       (5) Polarized light microscopic examination for crystals
       (6) Joint fluid glucose

3. The joint fluid must be examined promptly to avoid changes in the blood sugar or death of organisms.

4. If the joint fluid examination reveals a white blood count over 50,000 and/or a joint glucose 50 mg less than the blood glucose, the diagnosis of infectious arthritis is a strong possibility, but the tests in themselves are not diagnostic.

5. Antibiotic therapy is started before the results of the culture are known. Therefore, the initial antibiotic therapy is based on clinical judgment and is subject to change. The primary source of infection, the age, and occupation of the patient will influence your judgment. If you are guessing wildly, your best bet is penicillin G. However, modify your guess by the following knowledge: The penicillinase-resistant strain of staphylococci is increasing, particularly in the young and in the old. Therefore, in the infant up to six months of age and in patients over 40, start with a semisynthetic penicillin such as nafcillin. The commonest infection from six months to two years of age is H. influenzae, a gram-negative rod which is occasionally mistaken for a diplococcus. Ampicillin is the drug of choice for the infant from six months to two years of age. If cultures and smears are negative, repeat joint aspirations two to four times at frequent intervals (daily or less).

6. The antibiotics of choice if cultures are negative are nafcillin for the newborn to age six months; ampicillin, six months to two years; nafcillin, two to 14 years; penicillin, 15 to 39 years; nafcillin, over 40.[4] Coverage for gram-negative bacilli, for example gentamicin, should be included if the patient is immunologically compromised or the joint has prior damage.

7. Antibiotic therapy is accompanied by joint fluid aspiration and irrigation with sterile saline as often as needed to prevent joint fluid accumulation.

8. Failure to respond to therapy necessitates:

   a) A re-evaluation of the diagnosis
   b) A re-evaluation of sensitivity to the antibiotic, checking joint fluid for antibiotic activity
   c) Possible surgical intervention with drainage and tissue biopsy for smears and culture

REFERENCES

1. Parker, R.H. and Schmid, F.R.: Antibacterial activity of synovial fluid during therapy of septic arthritis. Arthritis and Rheumatism 14:96, 1971.

2. Owen, S., Jr.: Synovial fluid glucose. Journal of the American Medical Association 239:193, 1978.

3. Sommers, H.M.: The microbiology laboratory in the diagnosis of infectious arthritis. In: Clinics in Rheumatic Diseases. W.B. Saunders Co., Philadelphia, 1978, p. 63.

4. Clarke, J.T.: The antibiotic therapy of septic arthritis. In: Clinics in Rheumatic Diseases. W.B. Saunders Co., Philadelphia, 1978, p. 133.

5. Ward, J., et al.: The diagnosis and therapy of acute suppurative arthritis. Arthritis and Rheumatism 3:522, 1960.

6. Rytel, M.W.: Microbial detection in infectious arthritis. In: Clinics in Rheumatic Diseases. W.B. Saunders Co., Philadelphia, 1978, p. 83.

7. Layfer, L.F., et al.: Diagnosis of gonococcal arthritis by counter-immunoelectrophoresis: Detection of antigen and antibody in serum and synovial fluid. Arthritis and Rheumatism 21:572, 1978.

8. Brandt, K.D.: Gonococcal arthritis. Arthritis and Rheumatism 3:522, 1960.

9. Mitchell, W.S., et al.: Septic arthritis in patients with rheumatoid arthritis: A still under-diagnosed condition. Journal of Rheumatology 3:124, 1976.

10. Hermans, P.E.: General principles of antimicrobial therapy. Mayo Clinic Proceedings 52:603, 1977.

11. Nelson, J.D.: Follow-up: The bacterial etiology and antibiotic management of septic arthritis in infants and children. Pediatrics 50:437, 1972.

12. Schmid, F.R.: Infectious arthritis. In: Rheumatic Diseases. Katz, W.A. (ed.), J.B. Lippincott Co., Philadelphia, 1977.

13. Goldenberg, D.L., et al.: Treatment of septic arthritis. Arthritis and Rheumatism 18:83, 1975.

14. Swezey, R.L. and Spiegel, T.M.: Nonantibiotic aspects of treatment in infectious arthritis. In: Clinics in Rheumatic Diseases. W.B. Saunders Co., Philadelphia, 1978, p. 133.

15. Handsfield, H.H., et al.: Treatment of gonococcal arthritis-dermatitis syndrome. Annals of Internal Medicine 84: 661, 1976.

16. Leftik, M.I., et al.: Penicillin-resistant gonococcal poly-arthritis. Journal of the American Medical Association 239: 134, 1978.

17. Hunger, G. and Dandy, D.: The natural history of a patient with an infected total hip replacement. Journal of Bone and Joint Surgery 59B:293, 1977.

18. Charnley, J.: Postoperative infection after total hip re-placement with special reference to air contamination in the operating room. Clinical Orthopedics and Related Research 87:167, 1972.

19. Sledge, C.B.: Surgery in infectious arthritis. In: Clinics in Rheumatic Diseases. W.B. Saunders Co., Philadelphia, 1978, p. 159.

CHAPTER 14: VIRAL ARTHRITIS

It has long been known that viral infections may be accompanied by arthritis. The clinical importance of this is that some of the common viral diseases such as hepatitis and rubella may be associated with arthritis and must be distinguished from other forms of rheumatic disease. The viral arthritides are self-limiting and leave no residual joint infection. There is a movement on foot today to consider viruses as possible etiologic agents in rheumatoid arthritis and/or lupus but at this time it has no clinical application.[1]

Recently a parent in Old Lyme, Connecticut, reported to the state health department that physicians had diagnosed 12 cases of juvenile rheumatoid arthritis in her community. That number is substantially higher than what might reasonably have been expected, and it alerted brilliant public health officials who described an epidemic of benign oligoarticular arthritis in children in three Connecticut communities.[3] This epidemic may represent a true infectious arthritis secondary to a virus. Arthritis has been reported with multiple viral infections including chickenpox, infectious mononucleosis, rubella vaccine, arboviruses, adenoviruses, and mumps.[4,5]

There is a high incidence of rubella arthritis in adult patients. The disease is almost always polyarticular and symmetrical. It may be associated with fever and rash. The arthritis follows the rash after one to seven days and commonly involves the metacarpophalangeal and proximal interphalangeal joints of the hands (MCP and PIP joints). The arthritis seldom lasts longer than two weeks and leaves no residua. Hepatitis B (serum hepatitis) is frequently accompanied by arthritis. About half the patients with hepatitis B may have arthralgias. The syndrome of malaise, fever, anorexia, rash, and arthritis may appear long before the hepatitis is clinically evident. It is usually a symmetrical arthritis involving the small joints of the hands, knees, ankles, shoulders, wrists, and the joints of the feet. Patients may be quite ill with this type of arthritis; and because there may be false positive RA and anti-ANA tests and because there may be a decrease in serum complement during this period, these patients may be misdiagnosed as an atypical form of rheumatoid arthritis or systemic lupus. The ultimate diagnosis depends on the clinical course, the presence of a positive test for hepatitis B antigen which occurs in about 80 percent of such patients, abnormal liver function tests, and ultimately the development of icterus. Some of these patients, however, never do develop icterus.

Serum hepatitis as we know it today is a usually self-limiting disease. Time usually establishes the diagnosis and there are no known residual joint damages.

REFERENCES

1. Bennett, C.J.: Further research directions: The infectious etiology of rheumatoid arthritis: New considerations. Arthritis and Rheumatism 21:531, 1978.

2. Kaslow, R.A.: New England's own arthritis. Journal of the American Medical Association 238:330, 1977.

3. Steere, A.C., et al.: An epidemic of oligoarticular arthritis in children and adults in three Connecticut communities. Arthritis and Rheumatism 20:7, 1977.

4. Van H. Sauter, S. and Utsinger, P.D.: Viral arthritis. In: Clinics in Rheumatic Diseases. W.B. Saunders Co., Philadelphia, p. 225, 1978.

5. Mikkelsen, W.M., et al.: Twenty-first rheumatism review. Arthritis and Rheumatism 17:655, 1974.

CHAPTER 15: POLYMYALGIA RHEUMATICA AND TEMPORAL ARTERITIS

By Richard Rosenbaum

Polymyalgia rheumatica and temporal arteritis are aspects of an idiopathic systemic inflammatory disease. Excellent recent reviews are available.[1,2] Understanding the clinical aspects of the disease is essential to a discussion of therapy.

The disease may present with a number of different clinical manifestations. Patients may complain of pain and stiffness in muscles, particularly proximally, associated with morning stiffness and gelling. Symptoms are usually symmetrical. Systemic symptoms, including fever, weight loss, anorexia, fatigue, and depression are common. Giant cell arteritis most commonly involves temporal arteries with symptoms of headache or sudden visual difficulty. Arteritis in other large or medium-size vessels may become evident in the form of jaw cramping, intermittent extremity claudication, Reynaud's phenomenon, aortic disease, or ischemic mononeuropathy. Occasionally patients will have transient joint swelling. The disease may present with a distinct onset or appear insidiously.

Epidemiologically,[3] the patients are usually more than 50 years old. Males are twice as commonly involved as females. Incidence appears to be highest in Caucasians.

An elevated erythrocyte sedimentation rate is almost invariably present. However, occasional patients will present serious symptoms of the disease with a normal sedimentation rate, particularly early in the course of the disease. Other findings on laboratory evaluation may include a mild anemia with the characteristics of the anemia of chronic disease, a normal or slightly elevated white blood cell count, a rheumatoid factor in the blood of a few percent of the patients (this incidence is approximately equal to that of asymptomatic age match controls), a negative L.E. cell prep and ANA test, and occasional abnormalities of liver function tests, particularly an elevation of the alkaline phosphatase.

Although the disease is called polymyalgia and patients often complain of weakness, careful clinical testing rarely demonstrates motor difficulty that cannot be explained by pain and stiffness. EMG and muscle enzymes are normal, and muscle biopsy is normal or may show a mild, nonspecific atrophy of type 2 muscle fibers.

Arteritis changes in temporal artery biopsy are pathognomonic of the disease but are not invariably present. Pathologic changes include a round cell infiltrate in the media, fragmentation of the internal elastic lamina, intimal fibrosis, and the presence of giant cells. It appears that the pathologic lesion is not continuous in the artery. Therefore, one should follow the following biopsy procedure:[4]

1. Obtain a 3 to 7 cm section of one temporal artery.
2. Study the artery by frozen section.
3. Biopsy the contralateral temporal artery if multiple frozen sections of the first are negative.
4. Study multiple sections of both arteries if initial sections fail to show definitive evidence of disease.

Although some patients will have clinically abnormal arteries, many arteries that are normal to palpation will have characteristic pathologic changes.

Many patients will present with nonspecific myalgias and arthralgias or with systemic symptoms without evidence of arteritis. The laboratory manifestations are nonspecific, and the differential diagnosis in these patients often includes early rheumatoid arthritis, occult malignancy, sarcoidosis, or infectious diseases, such as granulomatous infections or subacute bacterial endocarditis.

In patients with evidence of arteritis, particularly in patients with visual difficulty, treatment of choice is prednisone or other corticosteroids. Initial dosage is approximately 45 mg of prednisone a day by mouth. One well designed study[5] suggests that 15 mg every eight hours or 45 mg every morning are equally effective. Both of these regimen appear superior to 90 mg every other morning.

Many authorities regard headache or a positive temporal artery biopsy in the presence of polymyalgic symptoms as evidence of severe arteritis. Some recommend treating such patients with moderately high steroid dosage such as 45 mg a day. This high

dosage is recommended on the assumption that such patients are
at increased risk for sudden blindness. We are more conservative about the use of large doses of steroids and treat patients
without clinical arteritic symptoms with an initial prednisone
dosage of 10 mg by mouth daily, slowly increasing the dosage
until symptoms are controlled and sedimentation rate has fallen.

Some patients present with polymyalgia or systemic symptoms
without clinical arteritis and with negative temporal artery biopsies. In these patients the diagnosis must rest solely on clinical grounds. If we treat these patients with steroids, we start
with 10 mg daily by mouth. Failure to improve after one or two
weeks of therapy is unusual in polymyalgia rheumatica. Of
course, the other inflammatory diseases included in the differential diagnosis may also improve on prednisone therapy.
Treatment of polymyalgia in the absence of evidence of arteritis with nonsteroidal anti-inflammatory drugs is occasionally successful.

There are no convincing data that define the proper time course
of therapy. Our policy is to continue initial prednisone dosage
for approximately one month or until the patient shows good
clinical improvement. A gradual taper of prednisone dosage
over a period of many weeks is then attempted. If symptoms
recur, steroid dosage is increased slightly. Some authorities
feel that a minimum course of therapy of one year or longer is
necessary in the presence of arteritis in order to prevent such
catastrophes as sudden blindness. Although we are constantly
aware of this threat, we prefer to use the patient's clinical status and his sedimentation rates as guides to tapering steroid
therapy. Our feelings in this regard are biased by seeing a
clinical population in whom polymyalgic symptoms are common
and steroid toxicity is seen frequently, but in whom arteritic
complications are relatively rare.

REFERENCES

1. Healey, L.A. and Wilske, K.R.: Manifestations of giant
    cell arteritis. Medical Clinics of North America 61:261-
    270, 1977.

2. Hamilton, C.R., Jr., et al.: Giant cell arteritis: Includ-
    ing temporal arteritis and polymyalgia rheumatica. Medi-
    cine 50:1-27, 1971.

3. Huston, K.A., et al.: Temporal arteritis. Annals of In-
    ternal Medicine 88:162-167, 1978.

4. Klein, R.G., et al.: Skip lesions in temporal arteritis. Mayo Clinic Procedures 51:504-510, 1976.

5. Hunder, G.G., et al.: Daily and alternate-day corticosteroid regimens in treatment of giant cell arteritis. Annals of Internal Medicine 82:613-618, 1975.

CHAPTER 16:   POLYMYOSITIS AND DERMATOMYOSITIS

By Richard Rosenbaum

INTRODUCTION

Polymyositis and dermatomyositis are forms of subacute inflammatory disease of muscles. The disease is characterized by gradual onset of symmetrical weakness, particularly affecting proximal muscles.

Presenting symptoms may also include arthralgias, distal weakness, Raynaud's phenomenon, sclerodactyly, myalgias, and dysphagia. Less common complaints are fever, weight loss, pulmonary or gastrointestinal symptoms, and calcinosis. An occasional patient develops EKG abnormalities or clinical arrhythmias.

In the case of dermatomyositis, the disease is accompanied by a characteristic skin rash. Recent clinical series[1,2] and a somewhat iconoclastic review[3] are available in the literature.

Serum muscle enzymes, electromyography (EMG), and muscle biopsy are indispensable in the diagnosis of polymyositis and dermatomyositis.

Muscle enzymes such as LDH, SGOT, CPK, and aldolase are usually increased, with CPK and aldolase being the most sensitive indicators of the disease. The electromyogram is usually abnormal. Muscle biopsy is often diagnostic.

The immune mechanisms involved in the disease and their role in its pathogenesis remain unclear.

Clinical varieties of the disease include pure polymyositis, dermatomyositis, myositis in childhood, myositis associated with malignancy, and myositis associated with collagen vascular diseases. The relationship between myositis and malignancy is not clearly defined.[4] Numerous series report increased incidence of malignancy in patients with myositis. Signs of neuromuscular disease may precede evidence of malignancy by many months or

may appear following diagnosis of malignancy. Myositis associated with malignancy does not have clinically distinctive features, except that patients with malignancy tend to be older and
to have a higher mortality rate. Although the exact relationship
between malignancy and myositis remains ill-defined, many authorities recommend an evaluation for occult malignancy in all
adult myositis patients.

Among the collagen diseases, myositis is most commonly associated with scleroderma but may also have overlap characteristics with systemic lupus or with rheumatoid arthritis. Patients
in this overlap category tend to be slightly younger and are more
frequently female than other polymyositis and dermatomyositis
patients.

DIAGNOSTIC PROBLEMS

None of the features of polymyositis and dermatomyositis is pathognomonic. For example, symmetrical proximal weakness of
subacute onset can occur in a number of other diseases, including some forms of muscular dystrophy, metabolic and endocrine
myopathies, toxic myopathies, disorders of neuromuscular trans-
mission, and infectious and granulomatous myositises. Con-
versely, on rare occasions a patient will present with other characteristics of dermatomyositis before clinical weakness can be
clearly demonstrated.

Muscle enzymes are a sensitive indicator of the disease, and
the CPK and aldolase will be elevated in the vast majority of patients. However, occasional patients will have normal enzymes
at the time of presentation. Furthermore, muscle enzymes may
be elevated in a number of other diseases associated with proximal weakness.

The electromyographic findings characteristic of polymyositis
and dermatomyositis include brief, small, polyphasic, easily
recruitable motor units and increased spontaneous activity such
as fibrillations, positive sharp waves, and bizarre repetitive
discharges. The electromyogram will be abnormal in as many
as 90 percent of patients with the disease, particularly if multiple muscles are sampled. Again, occasional patients with polymyositis or dermatomyositis will have normal EMGs, and the
EMG findings are not specific to the diagnosis.

A muscle biopsy, preferably with histochemical frozen section
techniques, is indispensable in the diagnosis of polymyositis or
dermatomyositis. In Devere and Bradley's series, 65 percent
had perivascular and interstitial inflammatory cell infiltrates

with or without muscle fiber degeneration and regeneration.[1] However, 17 percent of patients had normal biopsies and another 19 percent of patients had abnormal biopsies without changes that were definitely diagnostic.

Muscle biopsy should not be performed on a muscle that has been sampled for electromyography, because the EMG needle can lead to inflammatory changes. In patients with suspected poly-myositis, one should try to confine the EMG sampling to one side of the body and to choose for muscle biopsy a proximal muscle with moderate weakness contralateral to a muscle with demonstrated electromyographic abnormality.

Even if muscle biopsy is normal or nonspecifically abnormal, the biopsy is helpful in excluding some items in the differential diagnosis, such as lipid storage diseases.

TREATMENT

There is a paucity of data on the natural history of untreated polymyositis and dermatomyositis. Furthermore, treatment studies using well controlled experimental designs are lacking. Therefore, modern treatment of these diseases is based more on custom and consensus than on solid scientific data.

Good supportive care is essential to all patients. Dysphagia can lead to aspiration. Swallowing function should be monitored. When swallowing function is severely compromised, adjust diet or resort to nasogastric feeding or other means of alimentation. Respiratory distress can occur as a consequence of both respiratory muscle dysfunction and pulmonary fibrosis. Monitoring pulmonary function and blood gases is therefore important.

Patients with polymyositis and dermatomyositis readily develop contractures, and these can often be prevented by daily physical therapy concentrating on passively moving joints through their full range of motion. Aggressive physical therapy can often improve range of motion at joints already showing contracture. However, prevention is much preferred to correction of existing contractures.

The exact protocol for drug therapy is far from clear. Steroids are widely used in treatment of the disease, even though their efficacy is occasionally questioned[5] and has not been rigorously proven. A recommended practice is to begin therapy with 50 to 75 mg of prednisone daily or 100 to 150 mg of prednisone as a single morning dose every other day.[6] The relative efficacies of daily versus alternate-day prednisone are not well established, but an every-other-day regimen seems to decrease cushingoid side effects. In patients started on daily therapy, try to switch to alternate-day therapy early in the treatment regimen. On these high steroid dosages, serum muscle enzymes should begin to fall within the first month and clinical improvement in muscle strength should occur, usually within the first three to four months. After three months or more of therapy, as the patient appears to be making steady improvement, begin a slow tapering of steroid dosage. A typical regimen decreases the every-other-day steroid dosage by no more than 5 mg every three to four weeks. At the first sign of increased disease activity, steroid dosage is stabilized or slightly increased. As the steroid dose decreases, the rate of taper is also decreased. For example, once the dosage has been reduced to 50 mg prednisone every other day, dosage is decreased by only 2.5 mg a month. This slow taper commits the patient to two years or more of steroid therapy. Conceivably, a more rapid taper could be achieved in some patients. However, even with the gradual reduction in dosage suggested here, many patients will experience recurrence of disease activity as low dosage levels are approached. Some patients appear to require chronic low-dose prednisone therapy.

In patients who do not respond to alternate-day prednisone, one approach is to use daily prednisone or higher prednisone dosages such as 200 mg every other day. Alternatively, immunosuppressive therapy may be considered. A number of immunosuppressants have been tried. The most extensive published experience appears to be with methotrexate.[7] Because of the toxic nature of these medications and their unproven value, they should be reserved for difficult cases.

Many patients with dermatomyositis or polymyositis develop chronic muscle weakness despite therapy. In these patients with chronic weakness, it is very difficult to determine whether increased steroid dosage or addition of immunosuppressant therapy might lead to improved strength. An alternative possibility to be considered is that part of the weakness represents a steroid-induced myopathy. More aggressive drug treatment should not be undertaken in these patients unless muscle enzymes, a repeat muscle biopsy, or EMG give strong evidence to suggest active inflammatory disease.

Interpretation of status of patients during therapy is best done on clinical grounds. The patient should be followed using well-defined functional criteria of the muscle strength. Numerical rating scales, such as the widely used Medical Research Council scale of five, are hard to reproduce and re-evaluate on serial examinations. In addition, significant clinical changes in strength may occur without change in the MRC rating. Accordingly, evidence of functional ability, such as the patient's ability to rise from a chair, use his arms, or perform other activities with weak muscles, should be recorded.

It is important to emphasize these aspects of clinical examination because muscle enzymes, EMG, and muscle biopsy are much more difficult to follow and interpret. For example, it appears that steroids have a nonspecific CPK lowering effect in many muscle diseases and that a falling CPK may not be indicative of improvement in myopathy. Although, on statistical grounds, EMG abnormalities often disappear as disease improves, individual patients may improve clinically without changing their EMG or may show EMG improvement in the absence of clinical change. With muscle biopsy, serial evaluation is limited both by the sampling error inherent in biopsying a single muscle and by the impracticality of doing multiple biopsies.

Therapy of polymyositis and dermatomyositis requires long-term usage of high doses of highly toxic medications. It is therefore particularly important not to undertake therapy unless diagnosis is established as definitely as possible. Because of the diagnostic difficulties inherent in all of the diagnostic tests, do not undertake therapy without obtaining EMG, muscle enzymes, and muscle biopsy. When in doubt, consultation with one experienced in treating myositis is desirable before committing the patient to the rigors of prednisone or immunosuppressives.

REFERENCES

1. Devere, R. and Bradley, W.G.: Polymyositis: Its presentation, morbidity and mortality. Brain 98:637-666, 1975.

2. Bohan, A., et al.: A computer-assisted analysis of 153 patients with polymyositis and dermatomyositis. Medicine 56: 255-286, 1977.

3. Bohan, A. and Peters, J.B.: Polymyositis and dermatomyositis. The New England Journal of Medicine 292:344-347, 403-407, 1975.

4. Barnes, B.E.: Dermatomyositis and malignancy. Annals of Internal Medicine 84:68-76, 1976.

5. Mulder, D.W., et al.: Steroid therapy in patients with polymyositis and dermatomyositis. Annals of Internal Medicine 58:969-976, 1963.

6. Engel, W.K., et al.: High single-dose alternate-day prednisone in treatment of the dermatomyositis/polymyositis complex. Transactions of the American Neurological Association 272-275, 1972.

7. Metzger, A.L., et al.: Polymyositis and dermatomyositis: Combined methotrexate and corticosteroid therapy. Annals of Internal Medicine 81:182-189, 1974.

CHAPTER 17:   VASCULITIS AND POLYARTERITIS

"In the older patient with multisystem disease,
think of polyarteritis instead of systemic lupus."

Arthritis and vasculitis are important to the rheumatologist because of their association. Vasculitis may accompany the chronic
rheumatic diseases such as rheumatoid arthritis or lupus and
may be relatively benign; or it may be the primary disease, with
arthralgia being the presenting symptom. Because multiple systems are involved, the disease process may have protean manifestations, making its diagnosis elusive. Furthermore, the nomenclature used to classify vasculitis is confusing and is still
not universally accepted. One of the most useful categorizations
of vasculitis was achieved by Zeek[1] and later slightly modified
by Braverman.[2] This classification is largely based on histo-
logic differences and includes five divisions:

1.   Leukocytoclastic vasculitis is a term that refers to "nuclear
     dust," the destruction of nuclei seen in polymorphonuclear
     leukocytes which surround the vessel.[3] This type of vascu-
     litis occurs in systemic lupus erythematosus, rheumatoid
     arthritis, and allergic drug reactions.[4] Schonlein-Henoch
     purpura (HSP) manifests itself with arthralgis or objective
     evidence of joint disease.[5] The disease is characterized by
     a tetrad of purpura, hematuria, abdominal pain, and arthral-
     gia. It is not necessary that all four findings be present for
     the diagnosis to be made. The disease is more common in
     children than in adults; and, while the etiology is not proven,
     a drug reaction is frequently suspected. The disease tends
     to be self-limited and is usually diagnosed by biopsy. How-
     ever, in exceptional cases, renal involvement may be fatal.
     Treatment consists of removal of the offending drug and the
     use of steroids, although the latter's efficacy has not been
     unequivocally proven.

2.   Wegener's granulomatosis is characterized histologically by
     the formation of necrotizing granulomata in the tissues in

the vicinity of affected inflamed vessels. The disease usually starts as a severe upper respiratory tract infection with a sinusitis, followed by a persistent pneumonia and evidence of renal disease such as hematuria, pyuria, casts, and elevated urea nitrogen. Over half the patients have arthralgia, but frank arthritis is rare. The granulomatous lesion may even involve the nasal septum, giving the appearance of a saddle nose, suggesting congenital syphilis. The radiograph of the lungs shows nodules which go on rapidly to cavitation. The diagnosis can be made by biopsy of the nasal mucosa, lungs, or kidney, depending on the involvement of these organs.[6] The recognition of Wegener's granulomatosis is important because it has been reported that it responds well to the combination of cyclophosphamide and prednisone.

3.   Polyarteritis nodosa was at one time termed periarteritis nodosa. It is one of the most difficult of all medical diagnoses because of its variable presentations. The onset may be marked by nonspecific symptoms, including malaise, fever, and fatigue. Arthralgias are common, but frank synovitis rarely develops.[7,8] Eventually, the disease may involve multiple organs, including the kidney, the liver, the lungs, the skin, the intestines, and the peripheral nerves. The diagnosis should be confirmed by biopsy, but it is often suggested by the demonstration of tiny aneurysms seen with angiography.[9] The etiology of this disease remains controversial. The causes may be multiple. However, the demonstration that 30 to 40 percent of these patients have hepatitis B surface antigen in the serum and that this antigen can be found in vessel walls[10] has lent support to the idea that immune complexes are responsible for vessel damage. No treatment has been shown to be unequivocally of value in this disease, but steroids do provide symptomatic relief, and immunosuppressives are often tried. In many ways, this disease resembles systemic lupus in that it is a systemic disease with multiple organ involvement, resulting in bizarre symptoms. However, unlike systemic lupus which is primarily a disease of young women, this appears to be primarily a disease of the older male. One important clue is the presence of eosinophilia in the differential blood count. In suspicious cases, biopsies are essential. It is probable that the vast majority of these cases go undiagnosed.

4.   Giant cell arteritis is a form of vasculitis which may occur independently or may be a complication of polymyalgia rheumatica (see Part Two, Chapter 15, Polymyalgia Rheumatica).

5. Takayasu's arteritis is a very rare form of arteritis, at one time thought to be limited to oriental women. It still is reported to be a disease primarily of the female, 90 percent of the cases occurring in women. It is also called pulseless disease, aortic arteritis, and aortic arch syndrome. It is characterized pathologically by involvement of the aortic arch with giant cell infiltration of the arterial wall and medial necrosis. Stenosis and narrowing of the arch result in absence of radial pulse. Clinical symptoms include arthralgic fever, fatigue, and vertigo. The most important physical finding is the diminution of peripheral pulses in the upper half of the body. Diagnosis is made by arteriogram. There is no specific therapy, although steroids have been tried.

Polyarteritis may manifest itself primarily as a nervous system disease. This has been recognized since the original descriptions by Kernohn and Woltam in 1938. The disease, with its protean manifestations, can affect both the peripheral and central nervous systems. Peripheral nerve involvement ranges from a mononeuropathy to diffuse symmetrical polyneuritis. Polyarteritis is a classical cause of mononeuritis multiplex with multiple major peripheral nerves involved, often in an asymmetrical manner. The sympathetic nerves can become affected, leading to such findings as change in pupillary size and light response. Central nervous system manifestations in the disease are somewhat less frequent than peripheral manifestations and tend to occur later. The initial symptom is often severe headache. The patient soon develops manifestations of an acute brain syndrome with marked changes in intellectual function and later alterations in consciousness. Thrombosis can occur in blood vessels and may cause brain stem infarcts. Similarly, because of aneurysmal changes in the various arteries, hemorrhages can occur, either intracerebrally or into the arachnoid space.

REFERENCES

1. Zeek, P.M.: Periarteritis nodosa and other forms of necrotizing angitis. The New England Journal of Medicine 248: 764, 1953.

2. Braverman, I.M.: Skin Signs of Systemic Disease. W.B. Saunders Co., Philadelphia, 1970.

3. Sams, W.M., et al.: Leukocytoclastic vasculitis. Archives of Dermatology 112:219, 1976.

4. Gairdner, D.: The Schonlein-Henoch syndrome (anaphylactoid purpura). Quartery Journal of Medicine 17:95, 1948.

5. Winkelmann, R.K. and Ditto, W.B.: Cutaneous and visceral syndromes of necrotizing or "allergic" angiitis: A study of 38 cases. Medicine 43:59-89, 1964.

6. Wolff, S.M., et al.: Wegener's granulomatosis. Annals of Internal Medicine 81:513, 1974.

7. Nuzum, J. and Nuzum, J.: Polyarteritis nodosa. A.M.A. Archives of Internal Medicine 94:942, 1954.

8. Dollery, C.T.: Polyarteritis nodosa. British Medical Journal 1:827, 1969.

9. The enigma of periarteritis nodosa. Medical staff conference. Western Journal of Medicine 122:310, 1975.

10. Gocke, D.J.: Extrahepatic manifestations of viral hepatitis. American Journal of Medical Science 270:49, 1975.

CHAPTER 18:   SJOGREN'S SYNDROME

The term "Sjogren's syndrome" originally referred to a combination of dry eyes, dry mouth, and rheumatoid arthritis.[1,2]

It is now recognized that the symptoms of dry eyes and dry mouth may be associated with any of the connective tissue diseases - rheumatoid arthritis, systemic lupus, scleroderma, dermatomyositis, and polyarteritis nodosa.   Nevertheless, the term Sjogren's syndrome persists.[3]

Not all features of the syndrome occur simultaneously.   When dry eyes only occur, it is known as keratoconjunctivitis sicca;[4] when the predominant symptom is salivary gland involvement with enlargement of the parotid gland, it may be called Mikulicz's syndrome.[5]   The dry mouth symptom is termed xerostomia, and the combination of dry eyes and dry mouth is referred to as sicca complex.[6]

Today Sjogren's syndrome is thought of as a multisystem disease which may affect almost any organ or tissue.[7-9]

It is of importance to the rheumatologist because of its high incidence in rheumatic disease and because the symptoms, although possibly unrecognizably mild, may result in serious visual impairment.[10,11]

If Sjogren's syndrome is considered a separate disease, over half the patients have an associated rheumatoid arthritis, a large percentage have only the sicca syndrome, and the remainder are associated with other "autoimmune diseases."

Pathologically, the disease is characterized by an intensive lymphocytic attack on target organs such as the salivary gland, lacrimal glands, and, in severe cases, major organs such as the lungs, liver, and kidneys.   The lymph nodes are frequently involved, in which case it may be difficult to distinguish between a reactive hyperplasia and a true malignancy.   Even if the malignancy is recognized, it may be difficult to type.[12]

The disease represents a classic model of an autoimmune disease. There is a lack of "self-recognition;" so the T and B lymphocytes infiltrate and destroy their own body organs. The disease appears in animal models such as the New Zealand mice which are bred to produce systemic lupus.[13] There is often a marked elevation of serum immune globulins. A number of non-specific antigen-antibody reactions have been demonstrated to be associated with the syndrome, including salivary duct antibody, thyroid antibody, spleen and calf thymus antibody, in addition to positive RA tests, positive LE and ANA tests, and antibodies to kidney, thyroid, liver, lymphocyte, and smooth muscle extracts.[14]

The clinical symptoms of keratoconjunctivitis sicca (dry eyes) range from mild burning and itching to severe symptoms of pain, visual disturbances, and photophobia. The dry mouth (xerostomia) may be mild or so severe that the patient sips water constantly, develops inability to swallow dry food, has rampant dental caries and fissuring of the corners of the mouth (cheilosis).[14-16] In addition to the involvement of the salivary and lacrimal glands, the liver, the reticuloendothelial system, and the kidneys may be involved.

In advanced cases the diagnosis is made by history. In borderline cases tearing can be measured by the Schirmer test. A 5 x 34 mm strip of filter paper is folded 3 mm from one end, the folded end is hooked on the lower eye lid and left in place for five minutes. The irritation causes lacrimation. The normal subject will wet the paper past 15 mm. If tears are decreased as in Sjogren's syndrome, the paper will be wet less than 5 mm. The ophthalmologist can lend additional help with a slit lamp examination and rose bengal stain of the cornea and conjunctiva.[17]

Biopsy of the rudimentary salivary glands along the lower lip avoids biopsy of the major salivary glands and establishes involvement of these glands and the diagnosis.[3]

The treatment is primarily symptomatic. Methyl cellulose drops (artificial tears) may be instilled as often as every half hour. Sips of water and petrolatum on the lips eases the dry mouth. Secondary staph infections of the eyes or salivary glands may manifest themselves as red eyes or swollen glands and can be serious complications. In such cases, the help of an ophthalmologist or otolaryngologist should be sought, and appropriate antibiotic therapy instituted.

SUMMARY

Sjogren's syndrome is an "autoimmune disease" frequently associated with rheumatoid arthritis or other collagen diseases, or it may be present as an individual organ involvement. It is characterized by dry eyes and dry mouth due to a lack of tears and saliva. Treatment is symptomatic.

REFERENCES

1. Sjogren, H.: Zur kennthis der keratoconjunctivitis sicca. Acta Ophthalmologica 2(Supplement):1, 1933.

2. Von Grosz, S.: Aetiologie und therapy der keratoconjunctivitis sicca. Klinische Monatsblatter Fur Augenheilkunde 97:472, 1936.

3. Bloch, K.J.: Sjogren's syndrome: Clinical, pathological and serological study of 62 cases. Medicine 44:187, 1965.

4. Sjogren, H. and Bloch, K.J.: Keratoconjunctivitis sicca and the Sjogren's syndrome. Survey of Ophthalmology 16: 145, 1971.

5. Morgan, W.S.: The probable systemic nature of Mikulicz's disease and its relation to Sjogren's syndrome. The New England Journal of Medicine 251:5, 1951.

6. Buhim, J.J., et al.: Clinical, pathologic, and serologic studies in Sjogren's syndrome. Annals of Internal Medicine 61:509, 1964.

7. Shearn, M.A.: Sjogren's Syndrome. W.B. Saunders Co., Philadelphia, 1971.

8. Whaley, K., et al.: Sjogren's syndrome: Clinical associations and immunological phenomena. Quarterly Journal of Medicine A42:279, 1973.

9. Whaley, K., et al.: Sjogren's syndrome: Clinical associations and immunological phenomena. Quarterly Journal of Medicine B42:513, 1973.

10. Bunnim, J.J.: Heberden's oration: A broader spectrum of Sjogren's syndrome and its pathogenetic implications. Annals of Rheumatic Disease 20:1, 1961.

11. Lenoch, et al.: The relation of Sjogren's syndrome to rheumatoid arthritis. Acta Rheumatologica Scandinavica 10:296, 1964.

12. Talal, et al.: Lymphadenopathy and Sjogren's syndrome. Clinics in Rheumatic Disease 3:421, W.B. Saunders Co. , Philadelphia, 1977.

13. Kessler, H.S. , et al.: Eye changes in autoimmune NZB and NZB x NZW mice: Comparison with Sjogren's syndrome. Archives of Ophthalmology 85:211, 1971.

14. Bloon, K.J. , et al.: Sjogren's syndrome. I. Serological reactions in patients with Sjogren's syndrome with and without rheumatoid arthritis. Arthritis and Rheumatology 3: 287, 1960.

15. Whaley, K.: Current aspects of Sjogren's syndrome. In: Modern Topics in Rheumatology. Year Book Medical Publishers, Chicago, 1976, p. 71.

16. Hollingworth, J.W.: Management of Rheumatoid Arthritis. Year Book Medical Publishers, Chicago, 1978, p. 163.

17. Hazelman, B.L.: Ocular complications of rheumatoid arthritis. Clinics in Rheumatic Diseases 3:501, W.B. Saunders Co. , Philadelphia, 1977.

CHAPTER 19: BEHCET'S SYNDROME

By James Rosenbaum

When Behcet, in 1937, first described the syndrome that now bears his name, he limited the findings to oral and genital ulcers and iritis.[1] Although mucosal ulcerations and eye pathology are still prominent findings, Behcet's syndrome is now considered to frequently include arthritis,[2,3] a wide range of neurologic abnormalities,[4] skin findings including erythema nodosum, thrombophlebitis, and intestinal disorders. The disease has a male predominance and seems to be most common in Japan and in Mediterranean countries. In Japan the disease is associated with HLA-B5.[5]

The diagnosis is made on the basis of clinical criteria; no laboratory abnormality is specific. Its low frequency in this country may reflect in part a lack of clinical recognition. Oral ulcers are probably the most common findings. These are painful and recurrent, resembling the common coldsore or aphthous ulcer. The genital lesions do not tend to be painful in the female.[6] Biopsy of the oral lesions suggests that the underlying pathology is a vasculitis,[6] the cause of which is not known.

Joint manifestations are present in up to three-quarters of all patients.[2] Typically, this is a nondeforming inflammatory arthritis with morning stiffness. The knee is the joint most frequently affected and effusions are common.

Corticosteroids have in general been the mainstay of treatment. Not all authorities agree that they have been efficacious but they generally provide symptomatic relief. Other treatments have included antineoplastic agents, transfusions, and transfer factor. Levamisol, a drug that seems to enhance cell-mediated immunity, may be useful especially for the oral ulcerations.[7] (Levamisol is an experimental drug and is available in this country for experimental use only, after obtaining permission from the FDA.)

REFERENCES

1. Chajck, T., et al.: Behcet's disease: Report of forty-one cases and a review of the literature. Medicine 54:179, 1975.

2. Mason, R.M., et al.: Behcet's syndrome with arthritis. Annals of Rheumatic Disease 28:95, 1969.

3. Zizic, T.M., et al.: The arthropathy of Behcet's disease. Johns Hopkins Medical Journal 136:243, 1975.

4. O'Duffy, J.D., et al.: Neurological involvement in seven patients with Behcet's disease. American Journal of Medicine 61:170, 1976.

5. Ohno, S., et al.: Specific histocompatibility antigens associated with Behcet's disease. American Journal of Ophthalmology 80:636, 1975.

6. O'Duffy, J.D., et al.: Behcet's disease: Report of ten cases' three new manifestations. Annals of Internal Medicine 75:561, 1971.

7. Lehner, T.: Progress report: Oral ulceration and Behcet's syndrome. Gut 18:491, 1977.

CHAPTER 20: AMYLOIDOSIS

By James Rosenbaum

Amyloidosis is a disease characterized by the infiltration of organs with a material that Virchow thought resembled starch,[1] hence the name amyloid. This "starch" is now known to be a protein. In the form of amyloid that accompanies multiple myeloma, the protein is a portion of an immunoglobulin light chain.[2] This is also true of the protein that accompanies "primary amyloid" which tends to involve tongue, heart, skeletomuscle, joint, skin, bone, and gastrointestinal tract.[3] Primary amyloid is so frequently associated with a plasma cell dyscrasia that it is now generally accepted that the amyloidosis that may accompany multiple myeloma and the so-called primary amyloid are actually the same entity. In the secondary form of amyloid which accompanies chronic disease such as rheumatoid arthritis, tuberculosis, or osteomyelitis,[1] the origin of the protein is unknown. Secondary amyloid tends to involve liver, spleen, kidney, and the adrenal.[3] Amyloid may also occur limited to one organ and in a familial form.[3]

The rheumatologist must be aware of the primary form because of its association with arthropathy, and the secondary form because of its association with any chronic disease such as rheumatoid arthritis.

Primary amyloid may present as arthritis which clinically may resemble rheumatoid arthritis.[4] The joint pains can antedate the evidence for a plasma cell dyscrasia by several years.[5] Rheumatoid factor may be present though less frequently than with rheumatoid arthritis. The age of onset is usually later than for true rheumatoid arthritis. Often, a clue to the diagnosis is provided by the examination of the synovial fluid.[4] Typically, the cell count is low as it might be in the case of trauma. Often, protein that can be identified as amyloid will be seen in the synovial fluid. Amyloid joint disease is typically symmetrical, involving the shoulders, the wrists, and the knees.[6] When it involves the shoulders, the patient may present with a characteristic shoulder pad sign,[7] individuals with massive rubbery hard shoulders that resemble the pads of a football player. Carpal tunnel syndrome is also frequent in the primary form of the disease.

At the Mayo Clinic, the disease most frequently associated with secondary amyloid has been rheumatoid arthritis.[1] The development of hepatosplenomegaly or proteinuria should alert the physician to the possibility of amyloid.

Diagnosis is made usually invasively by rectal biopsy.[1] When negative, biopsy of an involved organ, such as the kidney or other synovium, may be indicated if the disease is still suspected.

The treatment of secondary amyloid involves therapy of the underlying disease. If myeloma overtly accompanies amyloid, steroids and cytotoxic drugs are used. Some authorities also use these agents in the primary form of the disease even if myeloma cannot be documented. Colchicine may eventually be shown to have a role in amyloid therapy.[3] It appears to be beneficial in averting attacks of familial Mediterranean fever, a disease primarily seen in middle eastern countries and frequently associated with amyloid. Colchicine also seems to be useful in the animal models for amyloid in which disease is induced by casein injection. Since the drug has relatively little clinical toxicity, it merits a trial.

REFERENCES

1. Kyle, R.A., et al.: Amyloidosis: Review of 236 cases. Medicine 54:271, 1975.

2. Glenner, G.G., et al.: Amyloid fibril proteins: Proof of homology with immunoglobulin light chains by sequence analyses. Science 172:1150, 1971.

3. Franklin, E.C.: Amyloidosis. Bulletin on Rheumatic Disease 26:832, 1976.

4. Gordon, D.A., et al.: Amyloid arthritis simulating rheumatoid disease in five patients with multiple myeloma. American Journal of Medicine 55:142, 1973.

5. Zawadzki, Z.A., et al.: Rheumatoid arthritis dysproteinemic arthropathy and paraproteinemia. Arthritis and Rheumatism 12:555, 1969.

6. Wiernick, P.H., et al.: Amyloid joint disease. Medicine 51:465, 1972.

7. Katz, W.A., et al.: The shoulder-pad sign: A diagnostic feature of amyloid arthropathy. The New England Journal of Medicine 288:354, 1973.

CHAPTER 21:   NONARTICULAR RHEUMATISM

In the 4th edition of "Copeman's Textbook of the
Rheumatic Diseases," published in 1969, an entire chapter was devoted to fibrositis. In the 5th
edition, published in 1978, only one sentence was
devoted to this condition.

"If we ignore the problem, maybe it will go away."

Arthritis refers to pathologic involvement of joints.   Rheumatism refers to involvement of connective tissue anywhere in the
body - muscles, tendons, ligaments, or joints.   Nonarticular
rheumatism, therefore, implies muscle and tendon aching outside of the joints.

Every practicing physician is acquainted with the patient who
complains of muscle aching and pain that is extra-articular.   The
location of this pain can be variable. Some of these patients present themselves with the classic story of morning stiffness associated with many of the inflammatory connective tissue diseases. They describe the prodromal symptoms of pain and prolonged morning stiffness. They describe generalized muscle
aching pain and stiffness, involving the muscles of the neck. In
some patients, the pain may be localized to the low back.   In
others, it may be confined entirely to the upper back.   The frustrating thing about these patients is that there is no objective evidence of disease. Occasionally, on palpation, one discovers
tender areas - so-called "trigger points" - but this finding cannot be duplicated on the same patient by other observers.   All
laboratory tests, including routine blood and urine studies and
even the exotic agglutination tests, are normal. The radiographs
offer no help in diagnosis.

This condition was given the name fibrositis by Gowers in 1904
in the belief that there was an inflammatory reaction in the muscles. This view was reinforced by Stockman in 1920, when he
described excised fibrous nodules which exhibited changes characteristic of low-grade infection but whose cultures were sterile.[1]

The American Rheumatism Association, in its 1973 "Primer,"[2] points out that the term fibrositis or fibromyositis is used to describe a symptom complex commonly seen in clinical practice but not proven to involve an inflammatory process. The "Primer" stresses that the patient complains of pain and stiffness in the neck, the shoulder girdle, and the extremities, that there are areas of tenderness and ill-defined nodules but that the rest of the physical examination, the laboratory studies, and the roentgenograms are all negative.

As Copeman[1] points out, nonarticular rheumatic pain is common throughout the British Isles and most European countries, but, if we judge by the American literature, it has never been well recognized in the United States and is generally thought to be psychologic in origin or to be associated with chronic tension states.

The "Twenty-second Rheumatism Review" (1973-1974)[3] points out that, in the past, rheumatism reviews have devoted very few pages to a discussion of nonarticular rheumatism in spite of the fact that this disease is responsible for nearly 10 million days per year of incapacity among the insured population of Britain. As the editors point out, the cost in lost man-hours of working time to the United States economy each year must be staggering. Because there are no objective signs of disease, the syndrome is ill-defined, ill taught, poorly treated and underresearched.

We are therefore faced with the problem that one of the most common manifestations of rheumatic disease is of unknown etiology, unknown pathology, and unknown treatment. As a result, there is a tendency to attribute the illness to psychosomatic factors. However, there is a haunting suspicion among treating physicians that the disease is organic in nature.

Many techniques for treatment have been suggested, including local injection of local anesthetics, local injection of steroids, oral use of various analgesics and anti-inflammatory agents. None is consistently successful. The physiotherapist usually is the most successful in handling these patients.[4]

In their management, these patients require a very thorough workup to eliminate the possibility that one might be missing an early rheumatoid arthritis, polymyalgia rheumatica, or a metastatic malignancy.

These patients should be treated with reassurance, analgesics as needed, and frequent follow-up visits, both for their psycho-therapeutic effect and for the opportunity they provide to recheck the laboratory work and reobserve the patient. It is a most frustrating syndrome to treat.

REFERENCES

1. Copeman, W.S.: Nonarticular rheumatism. In: Textbook of the Rheumatic Diseases. Williams and Wilkins Co., Baltimore, 1969.

2. American Rheumatism Association: Primer on rheumatic diseases. Journal of the American Medical Association 5 (Supplement):661, 1973.

3. Twenty-second rheumatism review. Arthritis and Rheumatism 19 (Supplement):973, 1976.

4. Awad, E.A.: Interstitial myofibrositis: Hypothesis of the mechanism. Archives of Physical Medicine and Rehabilitation 54:449, 1973.

Part Three: AIDS TO DIAGNOSES AND THERAPY

CHAPTER 1:   LABORATORY TESTS

"When I told her that her laboratory tests showed
improvement, she snapped, 'I could care less,
it's how I feel that's important.'"

A diagnosis of arthritis should never be based on laboratory tests alone because the tests are nonspecific. They confirm the diagnosis or they may suggest a diagnosis in an obscure case. Every patient with a rheumatic disease deserves a complete history, physical examination, appropriate x-rays, and what are today considered standard laboratory tests.

What follows is a summary of some of these tests and what should pass the physician's mind in attempting to make a differential diagnosis and in evaluating the rheumatic patient.

HEMOGLOBIN, HEMATOCRIT, RED BLOOD CELL COUNT

Anemia is usually present in an inflammatory arthritis such as rheumatoid arthritis or systemic lupus. It is usually absent in osteoarthritis or systemic lupus. It is usually absent in osteoarthritis, gout, or scleroderma. Approximately 80 percent of the patients with rheumatoid arthritis will have a hemoglobin in the range of 10-11 grams. If the hemoglobin is below 10 grams, other causes should be considered.

A drop in the hemoglobin in a patient under treatment signals possibly a deterioration in the arthritis or the development of a complication.

URINALYSIS

Albuminuria occurs in systemic lupus, scleroderma, polyarteritis, Sjogren's syndrome and amyloidosis. It may also be secondary to the drugs, particularly gold and penicillamine. The presence of excessive amounts of white blood cells in the urine should alert the clinician to a cystitis or a pyelitis. This is a common complication in rheumatic diseases and it is particularly important to recognize this because it may be the cause for the patient's clinical deterioration. Treatment of this condition may avoid overuse of some of the more potent drugs. Red blood cells, when present in the urine, should suggest the possibility of arteritis, cystitis, drugs, renal stones, and necrotizing papillitis secondary to some of the drugs, particularly phenacetin. The description by the patient of having passed smoky urine in the past or the development of a smoky colored urine on standing should alert one to the diagnosis of ochronosis.

WHITE BLOOD CELL COUNT

The white blood cell count is normal in osteoarthritis, is usually normal or very slightly elevated in rheumatoid arthritis. When the white blood cell count is elevated, one should consider an intercurrent infection, particularly the possibility of a septic arthritis. When the white blood cell count is below 3,000, systemic lupus or a Felty's syndrome should be considered. Eosinophilia should alert one to the possibility of periarteritis, a parasitic infection, an allergic reaction, or a drug reaction.

SEDIMENTATION RATE

There are three standard ways of measuring sedimentation rate - the Wintrobe, the zeta, and the Westergren method. The physician should select one that he is most familiar with and stay with that method. Most physicians prefer the Westergren method. The test is nonspecific. A number of diseases can cause an elevated sedimentation rate. The importance to the rheumatologist is that it helps to separate the inflammatory from the noninflammatory types of rheumatic disease. It also serves as a rough index to measure the progress of the disease. The sedimentation rate is usually normal in osteoarthritis, elevated in rheumatoid arthritis or systemic lupus, slightly elevated in gouty arthritis, and a marked elevation in sedimentation rate accompanied by an anemia should suggest the possibility of polymyalgia rheumatica.

C-REACTIVE PROTEIN TEST (C-RP)

This test indirectly measures blood proteins and is positive under the same circumstances as those which cause an elevated sedimentation rate. It is much more difficult to do than the sedimentation test and therefore is not ordinarily performed as part of the routine examination. It is nonspecific, indicating tissue necrosis or inflammation. On occasion, it may be elevated in some patients with rheumatic fever who have normal erythrocyte sedimentation rates. It is also not influenced by anemia, congestive heart failure, and hyperglobulinemia, which may affect the sedimentation rate.

ANTISTREPTOLYSIN O TITER (ASO)

This measures the antibody response against group A Streptococcus. It is positive in 85 percent of the cases of active rheumatic fever and if it is normal in its initial test, it should be rechecked in a week or two. A rising ASO titer is strong evidence for a group A Streptococcus infection and rheumatic fever.

SEROLOGY TEST FOR SYPHILIS

The routine serology test performed for syphilis is a nonspecific test, and a false positive serology occurs in 20 percent of the patients with systemic lupus. The presence of a routine positive serology test in a patient with rheumatic disease indicates a need for more specific tests to determine whether or not the test is a true or false positive.

AGGLUTINATION TESTS

The agglutination tests (see chapters on specific diseases) suffer from their nonspecificity and the fact that they may be positive in the normal population. They, by themselves, are never diagnostic of a rheumatic disease. In addition, these are biologic tests; therefore, there is a variation in the materials used for performing the tests and standardization is difficult. The following are the usual agglutination tests used in the diagnosis of rheumatic disease.

RA TEST (Latex Agglutination Test)

A positive RA test, particularly a weakly positive RA test is of no diagnostic value. The older the patient, the greater the possibility that the RA test will be positive; also, a negative RA test does not rule out rheumatoid arthritis. The value of the test is that it helps to confirm the diagnosis of rheumatoid arthritis. The more strongly positive the test, the more likely the diagnosis. A negative test with classic symptoms of rheumatoid arthritis should alert the physician to consider other types of arthritis; however, in the majority of cases, other causes will not be found and the patient will simply be said to have sero-negative rheumatoid arthritis. At this time, there is no evidence that this carries a different prognosis or a different response to therapy than does the sero-positive rheumatoid arthritis. Other forms of inflammatory arthritis such as systemic lupus, scleroderma, and periarteritis have a high incidence of false positive RA tests.

THE FLUORESCENT ANTINUCLEAR ANTIBODY TEST (FANA)

The value of this test is that it is exceedingly sensitive but non-specific. Many false positives are common. It is, however, rare for a patient with active systemic lupus erythematosus to have a negative FANA test. False positives are common and the test may be positive in many other forms of inflammatory arthritis.

ANTI-DNA TEST

The anti-DNA test is said to be more specific than the fluorescent antibody test. Because of the variation in the DNA used, there is a variation in reports from different laboratories. To some extent the test is still in the experimental stage and is not routinely performed by some laboratories. It does have more specificity than the FANA test but is less sensitive, and patients have been known to have systemic lupus with a negative anti-DNA test. A rising anti-DNA test titer suggests the possibility of activation of the disease.

SERUM COMPLEMENT

The system of serum proteins called complement is involved in the inflammatory antigen antibody response of lupus. Total hemolytic complement (CH50) C3 and C4 assays provide crude measures of its activity. In patients with known lupus, the combination of rising anti-DNA titer and falling complement levels suggests active disease but other inflammatory diseases may also alter complement levels.

CREATININE CLEARANCE TEST

A creatinine clearance test is a relatively sensitive indicator of impaired renal function. It is of value in detecting changes in renal function in systemic lupus and scleroderma and may show changes even when there are no albumin or casts in the urine. It should be done at least once and preferably twice a year in patients with these diseases.

TWENTY-FOUR HOUR URINE URIC ACID EXCRETION TEST

This is a difficult test to interpret because the uric acid excretion is subject to many variables: activity, diet, drugs, etc. As a rough screening test, it can be used to determine if the patient is passing excessive amounts of uric acid in the urine (over a gram a day) and because of this, the patient might be particularly susceptible to the formation of uric acid stones. It has no diagnostic value in making a diagnosis of gout or gouty arthritis.

CHEMISTRY SCREEN

Now that a battery of chemical screenings is part of the routine general workup, abnormalities in the screen may suggest many possibilities to the physician considering rheumatic diseases. It is important to recognize that there is a certain percentage of laboratory errors and not to simply treat an abnormal test.

GLUCOSE

An elevated blood glucose should alert the doctor to the possibility of diabetes. A diabetic glucose tolerance curve is not unusual in gout, or when corticosteroids are being used. This is not a true diabetes. A true diabetes may be the cause of a peripheral neuritis, which in itself may be a factor in muscle and joint pain; or the absence of pain secondary to the neuritis may be a factor in the development of an osteoarthritis.

BUN

The blood urea nitrogen is elevated in a number of situations accompanying rheumatic diseases. In gastrointestinal bleeding, the urea nitrogen is elevated but the creatinine is normal. An elevated blood urea nitrogen may indicate serious renal damage which occurs in systemic lupus, scleroderma, periarteritis, Sjogren's syndrome, etc.

CREATININE

The serum creatinine, like the blood urea nitrogen, is an indication of renal impairment. It is elevated later than the blood urea nitrogen; therefore, an elevated creatinine indicates even more serious renal damage.

SODIUM, POTASSIUM, AND CHLORIDES

These salts are important to monitor when large doses of steroids are being given. Steroids cause sodium retention and potassium excretion.

URIC ACID

The uric acid may be elevated due to drugs. The normal uric acid does not rule out gouty arthritis, particularly in its early phases. An elevated uric acid does not make a diagnosis of gout or gouty arthritis. There are patients who have asymptomatic hyperuricemia and never require treatment (see Part Two, Chapter 1, Asymptomatic Hyperuricemia).

CALCIUM AND INORGANIC PHOSPHORUS

Elevated calcium and decreased phosphorus should alert the physician to the possibility of hyperparathyroidism or a metastatic malignancy or it may be secondary to drugs. These tests should be repeated before any decision as to therapy is made. A decrease in serum calcium and an elevated phosphorus suggest the need to look for hypoparathyroidism.

TOTAL PROTEINS AND ALBUMIN

In some of the inflammatory rheumatic diseases, rheumatoid arthritis and systemic lupus, there may be a decrease in the total proteins and a reversal of the albumin globulin ratio. When the serum electrophoresis is performed, a hypergammaglobulinemia is not an uncommon finding.

CHOLESTEROL AND TRIGLYCERIDES

Marked elevation of cholesterol and serum triglycerides may be the cause of muscle and joint pain, although these are exceedingly rare clinical situations.

ELEVATION OF TOTAL BILIRUBIN AND INDIRECT BILIRUBIN

Elevation of bilirubin alerts the physician to liver damage. One should consider hepatitis or a drug reaction. There may be a transient elevation suggesting hepatitis.

ALKALINE PHOSPHATASE

It is important when the alkaline phosphatase is elevated to determine whether or not it is a liver or bone fraction. If it is a bone fraction, one must consider metastatic malignancy and Paget's disease. If it is a liver fraction, in addition to the conditions described under bilirubin elevation, one can occasionally find an elevated alkaline phosphatase associated with polymyalgia rheumatica and rheumatoid arthritis.

ELEVATION OF THE LDH AND SGOT

These are nonspecific enzymes and indicate damage to the lungs, muscles, or liver. To be more specific, if these tests are elevated, one should determine an SGPT which would indicate liver damage and a CPK which would indicate muscle damage. If there is a marked elevation of these serum enzymes, one considers lung disease, liver disease, and a muscle disease, particularly polymyositis.

CHAPTER 2: JOINT FLUID ANALYSIS

Joint fluid analysis is a relatively simple technique that can be performed in the office setting now that disposable syringes are available. It often provides a solution to difficult diagnostic problems and can only be superseded by direct joint biopsy as a technique in offering objective evidence of disease. From a practical point of view, it is the only way to distinguish between gout and pseudogout and to detect the organism involved in infectious arthritis.

Numerous excellent monographs with helpful tables have been written on the subject.[1,2] The major drawback of joint fluid analysis is that some of the findings are not specific. Thus, although it is usually said that a count of over 50,000 white blood cells represents septic arthritis, patients with rheumatoid arthritis or with gout may on occasions also have white blood counts as high as 50,000 or 100,000. Nevertheless, there are certain easily remembered and helpful principles that one can bear in mind.

Although joint fluid is most frequently aspirated from the knee because of its accessibility, any swollen joint can be tapped.

The tap, of course, should be performed under aseptic conditions. Some of the fluid should be put in a test tube with a small amount of heparin or EDTA, as clotting occurs rapidly and may interfere with the white blood count. If for any reason septic arthritis is suspected, culture tubes should be available and smears should be taken (see Part Two, Chapter 13, Infectious Arthritis).

The following simple principles should be kept in mind:

1. A normal joint has such a small amount of fluid in it that the successful aspiration of joint fluid in itself is usually indicative of some pathology, particularly if more than 1 or 2 ccs are obtained.

2. Normal joint fluid is clear. If the fluid is grossly bloody and the tap has been easy, traumatic arthritis or a rare form of arthritis such as one secondary to hemophilia should be considered. Cloudy joint fluid is common in rheumatoid arthritis; fluid from a tophaceous gouty joint may appear milky white; and the fluid of septic arthritis may appear purulent and on rare occasions may have an odor.

3. The white cell count in normal joint fluid is usually less than 400 cells per cubic mm. In osteoarthritis, the count is usually less than 1,000 or 2,000 per cubic mm. In rheumatoid arthritis, the count varies from 5,000 to as high as 10,000, but the usual count is around 15,000, and a count over 50,000 is exceedingly rare. In gout, the count averages approximately 10,000 or 12,000 and may on rare occasions simulate the count of septic arthritis. In systemic lupus, the count is usually below 5,000. In septic arthritis, the count is often over 50,000 and into the 100,000 range. A differential count is valuable in that a differential count showing over 80 percent polys suggests septic arthritis.

4. Blood cultures and smears should be done whenever indicated.

5. A blood and joint fluid sugar is valuable, particularly when septic arthritis is suspected. In most forms of arthritis, there is very little difference between the blood sugar and the joint fluid sugar provided the material is tested promptly. In septic arthritis, there is usually a marked difference between the two sugars.

6. The fluid should be examined under polarized light microscopy for crystals.

Periodic re-examination of joint fluid may at times be helpful in determining a patient's response and in re-evaluating a diagnosis.

REFERENCES

1. Kling, D.H.: The Synovial Membrane and the Synovial Fluid. Medical Press, New York, 1938.

2. Ropes, M.W. and Bauer, W.: Synovial Fluid Changes in Joint Disease. Harvard University Press, Cambridge, MA, 1938.

3. Hollander, J.L., et al.: Synovianalysis: An aid in arthritis diagnoses. Bulletin on Rheumatic Diseases 12:263, 1961.

4. Currey, H.L.F.: Examination of synovial fluid. Clinics in Rheumatic Disease 2:149, W.B. Saunders Co., Philadelphia, 1976.

CHAPTER 3:   THE RADIOGRAPH

A roentgenographic examination is essential in arthritis. It is of importance in confirming the diagnosis and following the course of the disease. Although at times the radiologist may be the first to make the correct diagnosis, the roentgenogram is not usually diagnostic at the onset of the disease when the pathology is primarily in the soft tissues. A normal x-ray examination does not preclude the diagnosis of arthritis. A normal x-ray in a suspicious case is an indication for repeated films at a later date if symptoms persist. What follow are some broad guidelines for the clinician. They are not a substitute for consultation with the radiologist.

OSTEOARTHRITIS

In osteoarthritis, the initial pathology is in the cartilage, not visible on x-ray, and for this reason when the patient is most symptomatic the roentgenograms are negative.

Late in the disease when joint space narrowing has occurred and osteophytes and sclerosis are visible, the patient may be symptom-free. The x-ray findings in osteoarthritis do not relate to symptoms. The patient with a "horrible" back on x-ray may be asymptomatic.

X-ray findings in osteoarthritis as compared to rheumatoid arthritis may be compartmental. Thus, in the osteoarthritic knee, only the medial or lateral compartment may show degenerative changes, whereas in the rheumatoid knee, the entire joint may be involved. This is an important diagnostic point and may be important therapeutically, because compartmental diseases suggest osteotomy as the surgical procedure of choice (see Part Three, Chapter 6, Surgery in Arthritis).

RHEUMATOID ARTHRITIS

Although films early in the disease may not demonstrate bone involvement, they are important to record further progress of the disease and to record the soft tissue swelling which may objectively prove illness.

Since subluxation of the cervical vertebrae (atlas on axis) is a serious complication of rheumatoid arthritis, flexion and extension films of the cervical spine as a baseline should be taken at the time of the initial examination and repeated if suspicious symptoms develop.

Rheumatoid arthritis involves cartilage, tendon insertions and synovium. The x-ray changes are periarticular. If the changes are in the bone shaft, they probably are not due to rheumatoid arthritis.

RHEUMATOID SPONDYLITIS

The earliest x-ray changes are in the sacroiliac joint. They are not well visualized on the usual AP views and are not part of the routine back x-ray. They should be specifically ordered so that oblique views are taken. In spondylitis, the lower two-thirds of the joint is involved. The initial changes are sclerosis and erosion on the iliac side.

Another early radiologic sign is squaring of the lumbar vertebrae. Erosion of the upper and lower corners of the vertebrae gives the lumbar vertebrae a shortened, square appearance.

SCLERODERMA

The only good objective clue in some cases is x-ray of the fingers for calcification around the tips (the CREST syndrome) (see Part Two, Chapter 7, Scleroderma).

PSORIATIC ARTHRITIS

Roentgen abnormalities may be the most specific clue in distinguishing psoriatic arthritis from rheumatoid arthritis with psoriasis. In psoriatic arthritis, the distal end of the phalanx becomes sharpened like a pencil point, and the bone it contacts overgrows to form a cup. The appearance is described as pencilling and cupping.

PSEUDOGOUT

Calcification in cartilage is diagnostic and demands joint fluid aspiration for crystal examination to confirm the diagnosis.

OCHRONOSIS

This disease is rare, but the x-ray of the lumbar spine is al-most diagnostic. There is marked disc narrowing with calcification at multiple levels and no osteophyte formation.

OSTEOPOROSIS

Osteoporosis is a common cause of back pain in the elderly. It is almost entirely dependent on x-ray for diagnosis. Poor x-ray technique may cloud diagnosis.

RADIOISOTOPES

Although radioisotope scans have been reported to show early changes in the sacroiliac joints, they are easily overinterpreted. Bone scans are of particular value in detecting metastatic disease, but again beware of overinterpretation.

CHAPTER 4: PHYSIOTHERAPY

In the best of all worlds, the arthritic patient would receive daily physiotherapy. I have seen colleagues (Dr. A.C. Jones and Dr. Robert Rinehart) achieve excellent remission of many forms of rheumatic disease using only programs of rest and physiotherapy. The limiting factors are economics and the cooperation of the patient.

Whenever it is available, physiotherapy should be prescribed. If it does not cure, it at least offers comfort and prevention of deformities. The modern therapist is a trained professional and is best qualified to determine the modalities of therapy to be used.

The occupational therapist of today no longer concerns himself with teaching the patient how to make potholders. The new occupational therapist is valuable in instructing the patient in proper hand use and function and self-help devices. What follow are some general suggestions in ordering therapy.

Cervical traction is of value in cervical osteoarthritis. However, in acute situations, it is best delayed for a day or two until the acute process subsides.

Ultrasound is most valuable when superficial areas are involved, particularly the temporomandibular joints and the hands.

Paraffin baths are of considerable comfort to patients with hand involvement. The therapist can teach the patient how to continue the procedure at home.

The patient with ankylosing spondylitis should be instructed in breathing exercises and the maintenance of proper posture.

An acutely involved joint should not be used actively. The therapist can carry out passive motion and massage of the adjoining muscles to prevent atrophy. "Use of the joint prevents disability" is an old wives' tale. Overuse of an involved joint is destructive and is determined by the presence of pain and/or swelling following use. Involved joints must be used judiciously; weight-bearing should be avoided.

Exercising in a warm heated pool is an excellent means of self-therapy. It permits use of joints and development of muscles without putting weight on the joint. The pool should be heated, preferably to 90°, but should certainly never be cold. Exercise in cold pools results in muscle spasms and is self-defeating.

Some therapists are trained to use biofeedback and/or muscle relaxation to relieve muscle spasm distress. These are often worthwhile procedures.

The minimum effective therapy frequency is two sessions per week; the ideal frequency, particularly during acute episodes, is daily therapy. In chronic subdeltoid bursitis (frozen shoulder, adhesive capsulitis) and in the shoulder-hand syndrome, successful therapy may require as long as six months to a year.

The Arthritis and Rheumatism Foundation has available, at both local and national levels, excellent articles on self-help devices. Patients can obtain reprints directly, or the physician can obtain them for distribution to the patient.

CHAPTER 5:   APPLIANCES, BRACES AND SUCH

In the good old days, appliances and braces came from the orthopedic brace shop. Today, ready-made appliances are available at most surgical or orthopedic supply stores. They can be prescribed by any physician and expertly fitted by a trained technician. A brief discussion of some of these appliances follows.

Where cervical traction is needed, it is best for instruction to begin by a trained physiotherapist. The patient can buy a cervical sling and traction apparatus which fits on a pulley attached to the top of a door. The patient, instructed as to the proper amount of weight, can utilize traction at home.

Cervical collars are available in all sizes, shapes, and colors and are fitted to the individual patient where cervical support is needed, as in a cervical sprain, cervical osteoarthritis, and occasionally in the rheumatoid where cervical subluxation has occurred.

Cock-up splints of the hand are usually fitted with the hand in optimum relaxed position, most often in slight dorsiflexion. In carpal tunnel syndrome or impending subluxations in the rheumatoid, they may offer enough relief to avoid surgery.

An elbow support is available which does not permit total extension of the elbow. This can be an invaluable aid in treating difficult cases of olecranon bursitis.

Finger supports can be homemade, using tongue blades or small frozen dessert sticks. Splinting an inflamed finger at night may give considerable relief in osteoarthritis.

A variety of knee supports are available. The simple elastic support is not sufficiently firm to be useful, but an elastic knee support with hinged metal sides which may even be mail-ordered offers enough support to give comfort to some patients with osteoarthritis or rheumatoid arthritis. A better fitting knee support is offered by the surgical supply stores. This can be tailored to the individual's exact size and may vary from the simple

240

elastic knee support with hinged metal sides to a comfortably laced leather support with hinged metal sides.

For back support, a lumbrosacral sacroiliac belt, if worn consistently, offers considerable relief in low back sprain and pain. In the patient prone to develop low back sprain, it can be worn prophylactically before the patient engages in a hazardous occupation. Full back supports with stays can also be ordered and expertly fitted. These are of particular value in problems of osteoporosis and degenerative arthritis of the dorsal spine. Ankle supports exist where there is ankle involvement. These are of elastic material with stays and are comfortable and work well.

A properly used cane can remove a considerable amount of stress from a knee or a hip. It should be carried by the hand opposite the involved joint. A technician should instruct the patient on the proper gait while using a cane.

Crutches, of course, are of considerable value in taking stress off the lower extremity. However, they are of limited use in rheumatoid arthritis, because often hand involvement precludes their use. Even when there is no hand involvement, continued use by a patient with active rheumatoid arthritis can aggravate the disease in the shoulders. Use crutches with caution in rheumatoid arthritis.

In addition to crutches and canes, there are four-legged walking devices that can be used temporarily by the severely disabled patient.

Transverse bars properly applied by a shoemaker to low heeled shoes offer relief when there is metatarsal involvement in osteo- or rheumatoid arthritis.

Sponge rubber heel pads in shoes relieve painful heels.

CHAPTER 6:   SURGERY IN ARTHRITIS

A generation ago, the orthopedist treated the arthritic.   Then rheumatologists were few in number, and the generalist did his best to avoid treating the arthritic patient.   As the rheumatologist came on the scene, the orthopedist bowed out.   He could accomplish far more with traumatic and congenital problems where there was decent bone structure; the rewards for working with the rheumatic were poor.   With the development of the methylmethacrylate (bone cement) and the Charnley hip procedure for total joint replacement, [1] the orthopedist has returned.   He is a welcome addition to the team; he can do much, but he cannot perform miracles.   In a chronic progressing case, he should be involved at an early stage because, in addition to performing corrective surgery, he can be of considerable help with casts and braces.

Total hip replacement has been attempted since 1891.   The early surgeons used ivory ball and sockets fixed in place with nickel-plated steel screws and glue.   As time went on, various metals, Vitallium, stainless steel, and plastics were substituted for ivory. The prostheses were screwed or glued into place.   Problems arose due to friction and metal failure or, more often, to the loosening of the screws and glue.

Charnley's introduction of an acrylic cement which acted as a space filler and the use of Vitallium for the femoral head and plastic for a cup has revolutionized joint replacement. Thus far, there have been no reports of long-term ill effects from the use of the cement, and some of the original joint replacements are still stable. [2]

The modern total hip operation produces so satisfying and spectacular a result when successful that there is a tendency to advise it regularly.   However, the procedure should not be undertaken without consideration of the possible accompanying mortality and morbidity.   The major postoperative problems are thrombophlebitis or pulmonary embolism, septic arthritis which can occur as late as five years after the implant, and local calcification of the surrounding muscles which may inhibit movement. [3,4]

The long-term effect and life expectancy of joint replacement is not yet known. Theoretically, an artificial joint must have a limited life expectancy due either to friction with resulting mechanical failure of the opposing materials or to the eventual separation of the methylmethacrylate from the bone. Bone is a living substance which changes; the glue is inert. The interface ultimately has to separate.[5] Recognizing these problems, total hip replacement should be performed only when the pain is so acute that it cannot be relieved by usual, safer means; and the disability is so severe that the risk of the procedure is justified. Old age is not a contraindication to surgery. I have seen successful results in patients over 85 years old. Youth represents a relative contraindication because of the unknown life expectancy of the prosthetic replacement.

Total knee replacement is less secure than total hip surgery. The knee has a hinge joint and a rotary motion. The current artificial joints used in the knee act primarily as hinge joints. The artificial knee is still not perfected. Therefore, indications for a total knee replacement are more rigid than those for a total hip replacement. The operation should never be considered unless the disability is great enough to require external support for ambulation. The aged wheelchair patient who needs only to walk around the house will be delighted with a total knee replacement; the football player will not. At this time, no other artificial joint can be recommended except on an experimental basis. Currently, over 500 different joint replacements are available.[5]

The incidence of thrombophlebitis or pulmonary embolism is lessened by the prophylactic use of various anticoagulants, such as small doses of heparin or aspirin. The incidence of septic arthritis has been lessened by improvement in operating room techniques and pre- and postoperative use of antibiotics.[6]

Review the following points before considering total joint replacement:

1. Be sure the patient is motivated.

2. Be certain in the older age group that there are no complicating neurologic factors such as stroke or peripheral neuritis.

3. If anticoagulant therapy is contemplated, be certain that there are no bleeding sources, renal or gastrointestinal.

4. Do not mix drugs that complicate anticoagulant therapy, such as aspirin and Coumadin.

5. Carefully examine the patient and eradicate all sources of infection: skin, lungs, genitourinary system. The persistent presence of an infection is a contraindication to surgery because aseptic arthritis usually ends with a total joint fusion.

6. If the patient has been on steroids preoperatively, be sure they are continued in adequate doses through the period of surgery.

Synovectomy of the knees has been in use now for at least 80 years.[7] The experts are still uncertain as to its value. One is not encouraged to recommend the procedure by statistical evidence of a success rate of 53 percent after one year[8] and improvement limited to relief of pain after eight years.[9] As the experts cannot agree among themselves on the value of synovectomy, it does not seem rational to refer a patient for a synovectomy to a surgeon who may perform only a few a year. At this time, synovectomy of the knees should be left to those engaged in research. I personally have little enthusiasm for the procedure, which I consider only on rare occasions when there is good systemic control of the disease but a remaining chronic synovitis in the knees.

HAND SURGERY

Various prostheses have been introduced as artificial finger joints. For the most part they have been made of plastic, rubber, or metal. In actual use, they act not as joints but as flexible spacers. They are still very experimental; breakage, loosening, and secondary infection are among the numerous problems experienced.[10] In my opinion, the failure rate of artificial finger joints has been too high to recommend use in the ordinary patient.

A nodular thickening of a flexor tendon sheath or thickening of a tendon, either in the digit or in the palm, can cause a "triggering" or a locking of the affected finger. Surgical removal of the nodule from the tendon or sectioning of the diseased tendon sheath gives relief and may prevent further disability. Rupture of a tendon demands repair, the sooner, the better.[11] The role of synovectomy as a prophylaxis to prevent joint and tendon destruction in the hand is still not resolved.[10,11] I would suggest a conservative approach. Fusion of a thumb or of a wrist in optimal position usually offers a good functional result and has stood the test of time.[5,12] The carpal tunnel syndrome that does not respond to conservative management with cock-up splints can be helped by surgical freeing of the median nerve.

THE FOOT

The foot should be considered in two parts: the anterior, which usually involves the metatarsals; and the posterior, which involves the hind foot joints. Problems usually develop in the metatarsals. If the patient cannot be made comfortable by the use of metatarsal bars, pads, and fitted shoes, then forefoot arthroplasty, almost universally successful, should be recommended. If the problem is in the hind foot, arthrodesises of the three hind foot joints is an effective means of eliminating pain.[13]

OSTEOTOMY

In osteotomy, the surgeon removes a wedge of bone and realigns either the femur or the tibia, thus shifting the line of pressure on a joint. In osteoarthritis, where the degenerative changes may be limited to only one compartment of the knee or one segment of the hip, the shifting of the weight relieves the pain and prevents further deterioration in the involved site. Osteotomy is a reasonably safe procedure.[5,15,16] It is seldom indicated in rheumatoid arthritis where the destruction is not compartmentalized. In osteoarthritis, particularly in the younger age group, it may well be the procedure of choice. Osteotomy is a simpler and safer operation than total joint replacement but does not preclude later total joint replacement when the patient will be older and the prostheses will be improved.

There are hundreds of surgical procedures available today to the arthritic patient. Each patient presents an individual and unique problem. The surgical procedures discussed are the common ones. The orthopedist must utilize his skill and experience to decide which alternatives can be offered to a particular arthritic patient.

SUMMARY

Surgery in arthritis is of value in preventing future deformities and in correcting those deformities that have developed. What can be accomplished depends a great deal on the skill, interest, and experience of the operating surgeon. Total hip replacement is currently enjoying great popularity; however, it should be approached with caution. The younger the patient, the greater the long-term risk. Total knee replacement is still far from satisfactory and should be performed only when there are no other alternatives. Other total joint replacement is still in the experimental stage.

REFERENCES

1. Charnley, J.: Arthroplasty of the hips: A new operation. Lancet 2:1129, 1961.

2. Lambert, J.R.: Surgery of osteoarthritis of the hip. In: Clinics in Rheumatic Disease: Osteoarthrosis. W.B. Saunders Co., Philadelphia, 1976, p. 653.

3. Freeman, P.A., et al.: Total hip replacement in osteoarthrosis and polyarthritis. A statistical study of results. Clinical Orthopaedics 95:224, 1973.

4. Charnley, J.: Postoperative infection after total hip replacement with special reference to air contamination in the operating room. Clinical Orthopaedics and Related Research 106:99, 1975.

5. Hastings, D.E.: Joint replacement. Journal of Rheumatism 5:117, 1978.

6. Ericson, C., et al.: Cloxacillin in the prophylaxis of postoperative infections of the hip. Journal of Bone and Joint Surgery 55A:808, 1973.

7. Goldthwait, J.: Knee joint surgery for nontubercular conditions. Boston Medical and Surgical Journal 143:286, 1900.

8. Marmor, L.: Surgery of the rheumatoid knee. Synovectomy and debridement. Journal of Bone and Joint Surgery 55A: 535, 1973.

9. Goldie, I.F.: Synovectomy in rheumatoid arthritis: A general review and eight-year follow-up of synovectomy in 50 rheumatoid knee joints. Seminars in Arthritis and Rheumatism 3:219, 1974.

10. Jackson, I.T.: Surgery of the hand in rheumatoid arthritis. In: Clinics in Rheumatic Diseases. W.B. Saunders Co., Philadelphia, 1975, p. 401.

11. Stillman, J.S.: The role of orthopedic surgery in the rheumatic diseases. Bulletin of Rheumatic Diseases 20:568, 1969.

12. Millender, L.H. and Nalebuff, E.A.: Arthrodesis of the rheumatoid wrist. An evaluation of sixty patients and a

description of a different surgical technique.   Journal of Bone and Joint Surgery 55A:1026, 1973.

13. Cracchiolo, A.: Knee and foot surgery in rheumatoid arthritis. In: Clinics in Rheumatic Diseases. W.B. Saunders Co., Philadelphia, 1975, p. 383.

14. Couentry, M.B.: Osteotomy about the knee for degenerative and rheumatoid arthritis. Journal of Bone and Joint Surgery 55A:23, 1973.

15. Jackson, J.P., et al.: High tibial osteotomy for osteoarthritis of the knee. Journal of Bone and Joint Surgery 51: B88, 1969.

16. Pauwels, F.: The place of osteotomy in the operative management of osteoarthritis of the hip.   Triangle 8:196, 1967-1968.

Part Four: REVIEW

HELPFUL HINTS IN THE DIAGNOSIS AND
TREATMENT OF RHEUMATIC DISEASES

The patient with classic rheumatoid arthritis has bilateral, symmetrical, peripheral joint involvement, but the disease may also, at its onset, be monoarticular or may start with exacerbations and remissions resembling gout.

Prolonged morning stiffness is an extremely important symptom in rheumatoid arthritis. The patient volunteers that he is so stiff in the morning that he has difficulty getting out of bed and that he requires at least an hour to loosen up. Occasionally, when the disease has a milder onset, the stiffness may be limited to the hands. The patient may find it necessary to put his hands in warm water before he can begin the day.

Patients with rheumatoid arthritis are always worse in the morning. In milder cases, their joints may be swollen in the morning and normal by midday. Examine a patient with a questionable diagnosis early in the morning.

Never make a diagnosis of rheumatoid arthritis based on a positive RA blood test. Remember that the RA test may be positive in five percent of the normal population and higher in the older population.

A sero-negative RA test does not negate the diagnosis of rheumatoid arthritis when other appropriate signs and symptoms are present, but it does alert the physician to watch for other types of rheumatic disease that might mimic rheumatoid arthritis. In these patients, carefully examine the skin for psoriasis, review the gastrointestinal history and history of the onset of the illness.

Psoriatic arthritis may be associated with a minimal amount of psoriasis. The psoriasis may be limited to the nails or a slight patch around the hair or elbows. The sausage fingers, the involvement of the terminal phalangeal joints, and the x-ray changes are diagnostic.

Any arthritic with a history of rectal bleeding or gastrointestinal disturbances should have a proctoscopic and upper and lower gastrointestinal roentgenogram. Arthritis may precede granulomatous and ulcerative bowel disease by years. The bowel disease, when discovered, may be minimal.

Back pain, insidious at onset in a young male, persisting for more than three months, and associated with morning stiffness relieved by exercise, is strongly suggestive of spondylitis. When the patient is a reliable historian, the history is quite characteristic.[1]

The earliest physical sign of ankylosing spondylitis is decrease in chest expansion. Chest expansion in the normal patient should be greater than two inches.

The earliest radiologic sign in ankylosing spondylitis is bilateral sclerosis of the sacroiliac joints. Radioisotope bone scans of the joints, when properly interpreted, may be even more sensitive than the standard roentgenograms. The sacroiliac joint x-rays are not usually part of a standard lumbar spine x-ray examination and must be ordered specifically, when the standard A-P view is not diagnostic.

In the postmenopausal female complaining of chronic back pain, consider osteoporosis. Since the diagnosis depends entirely on radiographic studies which occur late in the disease, the disease is probably more often missed than diagnosed.

The patient with rheumatoid arthritis, except in a few rare instances, seldom has an elevated temperature. Such patients should be carefully examined for the possibility of a septic arthritis. Sources of infection, particularly the urine and the lungs, should be checked.

Although aspirin is considered the drug of choice in the treatment of rheumatoid arthritis, some patients may be sensitive to the drug and may actually be made worse by aspirin. Occasionally, ask the patient with the chronic disease to bring in all the medications that he is taking. You may be surprised at the size of the package brought in and amazed at the medications that are being taken and not taken.

In rheumatoid arthritis, doses of prednisone over 10 mg daily may actually cause muscle pain and aching.

In using steroids, it is much easier to start with a low dose and increase the dosage than to start with a high dose and decrease the dosage.

In withdrawing steroids, consider use of 1 mg tablets. Never be in a hurry to withdraw the steroids. Project at least six months to a year in withdrawal time. Lower the dosage only 1 mg every month and remember that even that 1 mg may have a critical effect upon the patient's illness.

A patient with chronic gouty arthritis may at times resemble the patient with rheumatoid arthritis. This is particularly true in the patient with gout that has been mistreated and misdiagnosed.

Gout and rheumatoid arthritis rarely coexist, but it does happen occasionally.

Rheumatoid arthritis is exceedingly rare in the psychotic.

In the patient with rheumatoid arthritis who has a white blood count less than 3,000, seriously consider the diagnosis of systemic lupus erythematosus.

The patient with rheumatoid arthritis who is doing poorly can sometimes be helped by three weeks of hospitalization.

One of the best diagnostic tests available is joint fluid examination. Do not neglect this procedure.

REFERENCE

1. Callan, A., et al.: Clinical history as a screening test for ankylosing spondylitis. Journal of the American Medical Association 237:2613, 1977.

SUMMARY OF RHEUMATIC DISEASES:
THEIR DIAGNOSIS AND TREATMENT

The bulk of the patients seen in office practice will have osteo-arthritis. This is primarily a disease of the older patient. It is not accompanied by any systemic symptoms. It is usually limited to one or two joints or localized in an area of the spine. Stiffness is present but is not a major symptom. This stiffness is usually of short duration. The major symptom is pain with use and pain persisting after use. There is often associated pain at rest and at night. Since the primary disease process is in the cartilage, when the disease starts the radiographs are usually normal. By the time the radiographic changes occur, the patient may be symptom-free. Laboratory tests are usually normal in this disease. A common problem is the postmeno-pausal woman who presents herself with swelling of the terminal phalangeal joints. This represents no diagnostic problem. In some cases, however, there may also be involvement of the proximal interphalangeal joints and the base of the thumb. This may present some difficulty in distinguishing it from rheumatoid arthritis. With the localized nature of the disease, the absence of other joint involvement, the normal laboratory tests, and the age of the patient are helpful in the differential diagnosis. Osteoarthritis is usually not a crippling disease unless the hip or the knee are involved and although it is not generally empha-sized, clinical experience indicates that the symptoms of pain are self-limiting, lasting possibly for a few years as the acute inflammatory initial process subsides and by the time the x-ray changes take place, the patient is often symptom-free. One of the major complications of the disease occurs when it is in the cervical or lumbar spine and then there may be nerve involve-ment which is much more difficult to relieve but seldom requires a surgical approach.

As for the treatment, many patients can be helped by simple re-assurance. Once they realize that the disease is not crippling and can be relieved by aspirin, they may require no further medi-cal help. If aspirin is not tolerated or does not relieve the symptoms, then the newer nonsteroidal anti-inflammatory agents should be tried. They have better patient acceptance, are easier to manage, but are more expensive. Indomethacin and phenyl-butazone are far more effective than aspirin or the newer anti-inflammatory agents but introduce the problem of greater toxi-city. Simple supporting devices such as a cervical collar, a lumbosacral belt with a sacroiliac support, knee supports, elas-tic with hinged metal sides, stiff ankle supports, an elbow cage, a cane, and crutches offer relief. Physiotherapy is always of help. Intra-articular, relatively insoluble forms of hydrocor-tisone are very effective in relieving the patient symptomatically and should be tried once or twice, but repeated injections are contraindicated because there is some suggestion that they may hasten cartilage degeneration if repeatedly used.

The second large group of patients seen in the office practice are patients with rheumatoid arthritis. This is usually a young woman with bilateral symmetrical involvement of the joints as-sociated with systemic symptoms of stiffness, night pain, weight loss, and even fever. It can affect any age group and may have an atypical onset and be mono- or oligoarticular in its initial presentation. It may also occasionally present itself with ex-acerbations and remissions. The morning stiffness, the swollen joints, the anemia, the elevated sedimentation rate, and the pos-itive RA test are all helpful in diagnosis. Every patient who pre-sents herself as having possible rheumatoid arthritis should be suspected as a patient with possible systemic lupus erythemato-sus. If the patient has albumin cells or casts in the urine, a white blood count below 3,000, a positive serology, evidence of multisystem disease, a history of drug or sun sensitivity, un-explained skin rashes, or alopecia, then systemic lupus should be strongly suspected. Every patient with rheumatoid arthritis then deserves to have at least a fluorescent antinuclear antibody test as a screening test and, where available, an anti-DNA test.

The treatment of rheumatoid arthritis is empiric and should be individualized. Because most physicians have learned of rheu-matoid arthritis in hospitalized patients, they have a distorted view of the natural history of the disease. Many patients in their initial onset, if treated conservatively, may go into a spontane-ous remission. Therefore, it is important, even in patients who may have a violent onset, that the initial therapy be extremely conservative. This should consist of a prescribed period of rest, physiotherapy, and aspirin given in regular doses to achieve a blood level of 20 mg percent. If aspirin does not work, then newer nonsteroidal anti-inflammatory agents are of value. The older anti-inflammatory agents such as indomethacin and phenyl-butazone work in a small percentage of cases but they do intro-duce the problem of toxicity.

If the disease shows progression under conservative management, then the physician must choose between the antimalarials
(chloroquine, hydroxychloroquine) or gold. The antimalarials
have the advantage that they can be taken by mouth and that they
produce results in 30 to 60 days. They have the disadvantage of
a reputation of possibly producing blindness due to retinal toxicity. Gold has stood the test of time. It is the one approved
drug that may in some cases actually produce a true remission.
It requires three to six months before it is effective, it must be
given peripherally, and there is a high incidence of toxicity and
even fatality. The patient on gold therapy should be carefully
monitored for skin rashes, stomatitis, thrombocytopenia, agranulocytosis, or an aplastic anemia. If the patient responds to
gold, the patient should be kept on maintenance gold therapy
for life.

Penicillamine is currently very popular in Great Britain. It may
be effective when gold fails. A new dosage schedule which recommends 250 mg daily for three months, and then increments
of 250 mg daily every three months until a total dosage of 1
gm daily is reached, has lessened toxicity. The drug must be
as carefully monitored as gold and does have a high incidence of
toxicity.

The immunosuppressives may produce dramatic results in some
patients. At this time, azathioprine is the current favorite because the ratio between efficacy and toxicity appears to be reasonable. Cyclophosphamide is probably the most effective but
is very toxic and should be used only in very desperate cases.
In actual practice, of the total number of patients with rheumatic
disease, only a very few have true indications for a trial with
the immunosuppressives.

The corticosteroids, usually given as prednisone, do produce
dramatic results. The major problem is when to introduce them
in the patient's therapy. Certainly, never as the initial drug.
In a few cases they almost seem to be specific. If the drug is
used, never exceed 7.5-10 mg. Alternate-day therapy has been
suggested to lessen toxicity but this does not work in rheumatoid
arthritis because on the off days, the patient is much worse.
These drugs are often used in conjunction with other drugs.
Once started they should never be stopped abruptly and the patient should carry identifying information on him, because if involved in an accident, extra doses must be given to prevent
shock.

Propoxyphene and acetaminophen are analgesic but not anti-inflammatory. They are commonly used by patients with rheumatic

disease because they produce less gastrointestinal disturbance; they do lack the anti-inflammatory effect of the other drugs.

The young male who presents himself with a story of chronic back pain should always be suspected of having ankylosing spondylitis. The important symptom is night pain and morning stiffness lasting for a long period of time and relieved by activity. The first important physical finding is decreased chest expansion, less than two inches. The earliest radiologic evidence of the disease is sclerosis of the sacroiliac joints. In borderline cases, tissue-typing is helpful because 90 percent of these patients are said to be HLA-B27 positive.

The patient with ankylosing spondylitis should be treated with a program of education as to posture and breathing, a trial of aspirin or the newer anti-inflammatory drugs. Indomethacin and phenylbutazone usually work dramatically in this disease and if they are not effective, the motivation or the diagnosis should be suspect.

The middle-aged male who presents himself with an acute painful peripheral monoarticular arthritis of sudden onset should be suspected of having gout. If there is a history of a previous attack with spontaneous remission, the probability that this is gout becomes very high. The characteristic gouty joint is extremely tender, extremely painful and erythematous, suggesting a cellulitis. The joint fluid aspiration should be performed if possible to verify the diagnosis and to eliminate pseudogout (chondrocalcinosis gout). The patient with an acute attack of gout will respond dramatically to indomethacin 50 mg four times a day or phenylbutazone, 200 mg four times a day, with a rapid reduction of dosage in both cases on the second day to a minimum maintenance dose. The uricosuria accompanying gout should not be treated until all acute symptoms have subsided. At that time the patient should be put on maintenance colchicine, 0.6 mg, one tablet twice a day, and a uricosuric agent added. This can be probenecid, sulfinpyrazone, or allopurinol.

The sexually active patient who presents himself with painful swollen joints, whether monoarticular or multiple, should be suspected of having a gonorrheal arthritis. A careful history should be taken to rule out Reiter's disease. The patient should be carefully examined and appropriate smears and cultures taken for gonorrhea; and joint fluid aspiration and culture should be performed to aid in the diagnosis. Appropriate antibiotic therapy should be instituted as soon as there is reasonable evidence that the antibiotic being used is the proper one.

Systemic lupus erythematosus was once considered a very rare disease. With the discovery of the L.E. cell by Hargraves, what was once a rare disease has now become relatively common. It is usually a disease of young women, and 75 percent of the patients present themselves with arthralgias so that it is difficult to distinguish them from the patients with rheumatoid arthritis. A large percentage of these patients are now known to have central nervous system involvement, and the initial presenting symptom may be a seizure, a psychosis, or a psychoneurosis. It is exceedingly difficult to make a diagnosis of systemic lupus in these patients in the absence of other system involvement. Any young woman who presents herself with arthralgia, multiple system diseases, or undiagnosed disease should be suspected as a possible patient with systemic lupus erythematosus. Helpful in the diagnosis are the laboratory tests, a fluorescent antinuclear antibody test, and an anti-DNA test. These tests in themselves, however, are not sufficient evidence on which to base a diagnosis nor does their absence exclude the diagnosis.

As the diagnosis of lupus has been expanded to include a large group, it has become evident that most of these patients who do not have renal or central nervous system involvement actually have a good prognosis, and spontaneous remissions may occur. In some patients the disease may be drug-induced. Simple cessation of the offending drug results in a cure. Other patients, even though the offending agent may be unknown, may go into spontaneous remission. Unless these patients present themselves with threatening symptoms, they should be treated extremely conservatively, even more conservatively than the patients with rheumatoid arthritis. Milder cases can be handled with reassurance and the nonsteroidal anti-inflammatory agents. Chloroquine, hydroxychloroquine and Atabrine seem to be extremely effective in these patients with arthralgia and skin manifestations. Gold is not used in this disease. Corticosteroids are indicated only when more conservative means fail; large doses of corticosteroids are indicated in life-threatening situations such as renal involvement, hemolytic anemia, thrombocytopenia, and central nervous system involvement. The value of immunosuppressives in this disease is unproven. A recent study indicated that only 25 percent of the experts use immunosuppressives. It is probably wise to consider the immunosuppressives as an experimental procedure that should be limited to scientific clinical investigation. Do not feel guilty if you do not put your patient on immunosuppressives. The argument that because the disease is fatal, a toxic drug is indicated is not very logical.

Scleroderma is an exceedingly rare disease. It presents a problem because in its initial onset, it may simulate rheumatoid arthritis. It is usually accompanied by normal laboratory tests. Its diagnosis in its initial onset is based purely on the history and physical examination. Skin biopsies at this stage are seldom of value. The treatment is unsatisfactory, nonspecific, and empiric.

Mixed connective tissue disease is a disease that resembles rheumatoid arthritis and is distinguished from it by specific antibody reactions. These patients agglutinate RNP in high titers. Some experts feel that mixed connective tissue disease is a variant of systemic lupus erythematosus.

Sjogren's syndrome is characterized by keratoconjunctivitis sicca, dry eyes, and xerostomia (dry mouth) in combination with an "autoimmune disease" such as rheumatoid arthritis. It may be so mild that it is never diagnosed or so severe that it leads to blindness and unquenchable thirst. The diagnosis is made by ophthalmologic tests, and by biopsy of the rudimentary salivary glands of the lip. The treatment is very unsatisfactory and is purely symptomatic.

There are a number of diseases that used to be classified as rheumatoid arthritis but have now been recognized as separate entities. These are rheumatoid spondylitis, psoriatic arthritis, Reiter's syndrome, and arthritis associated with enteritis. These diseases differ from rheumatoid arthritis in that they are RA negative, are atypical in their joint distribution and involvement. A large percentage of these cases are HLA-B27 positive and those patients that are HLA-B27 positive usually show evidence of spondylitis and sacroiliac involvement. These diseases are accompanied by the underlying disease which sometimes may be minimal. Thus psoriatic arthritis is accompanied by psoriasis, Reiter's syndrome, by urethritis and conjunctivitis, and the arthritis associated with enteritis is accompanied by Crohn's disease or ulcerative colitis. These patients seem to have a better prognosis than those patients with rheumatoid arthritis. The treatment of the underlying disease may often eliminate the peripheral arthritic component. The sacroiliitis usually responds well to the same drugs that are used in the treatment of rheumatoid spondylitis.

In office practice, there is a large subgroup of patients who receives scant attention in the literature. These are patients who are labeled as having fibrositis. These patients complain of stiffness, aching, and fatigue. At times their story may be very dramatic and may resemble the fibrositis that occurs in rheumatoid arthritis. The problem is that in these patients, all the laboratory tests are normal, muscle biopsies offer no help, and roentgenograms are not diagnostic. To make the matter worse, many of these patients do not respond to any of the drugs usually used in the treatment of rheumatic diseases. In the absence of objective evidence of disease, the physician is faced with the problem as to whether or not these patients have a psychogenic disease or have an organic disease which we have not been able to define. The physician who sees a number of these patients has a haunting fear that a great many of them are organic, but we simply have not found the diagnostic clue. At this time, they must each be treated individually. The patient that obviously has a psychogenic rheumatism should be treated as any patient with a psychosomatic illness. The patient in whom the physician suspects that the disease may be organic should be watched and monitored with repeated laboratory tests. A few of these patients may be in the prodromal stages of one of the inflammatory arthritides. There is no satisfactory treatment and no satisfactory answer at this time for this large group.

The promise by some physicians that early detection invariably results in a cure, the announcement of miracle drugs by the press, the perpetuation by the courts of the legal fiction that physicians should be infallible have given the public unreal expectations and made the treatment of a difficult disease even more complicated.

GLOSSARY: DRUGS AND THEIR USUAL DOSAGES

INTRODUCTION

This section outlines the usual dosages for the drugs referred to within the text. In most instances, the generic name is accompanied by some of its common trade names.

The fact that all trade names are not included does not imply that the ones omitted are of lesser quality than those indicated. Therefore, I have used the names with which I am familiar.

Because these drugs are in themselves toxic and are being used in a particularly susceptible patient population, and since knowledge of toxicity keeps changing, it is well to constantly review the package inserts before using a specific drug. Since patients with rheumatoid arthritis are very prone to be on multiple drugs, the problem of drug interaction is a constant hazard.

The dosage that is given is the usual maximum dose. There seems to be little point in most cases in exceeding the maximum dose. The general principle is that once the patient is comfortable, the dosage is reduced to the minimum effective dose. One should be alert to the fact that many of these drugs have not been tested in children or in lactating mothers or in pregnancy.

SALICYLATES

ASPIRIN USP
325 mg tablet

Aspirin is available in 65 mg, 81 mg, 162 mg, 325 mg, 500 mg, and 650 mg tablets. Over 200 forms are available.

ASCRIPTIN

Aspirin 325 mg mixed with magnesium aluminum hydroxide 150 mg

ASCRIPTIN A/D

Aspirin 325 mg, but the amount of magnesium aluminum hydroxide is double, 300 mg

ECOTRIN (Enteric-coated Aspirin)
325 mg tablet

SALSALATE (Disalcid) Also described as salicyl-salicylic acid

Each tablet contains 500 mg salsalate. Suggested adult dose is two tablets t.i.d.

CHOLINE MAGNESIUM TRISALICYLATE (Trilisate)
500 mg

Choline salicylate combined with magnesium salicylate. Dose one to three b.i.d.

::

NONSTEROIDAL ANTI-INFLAMMATORY AGENTS

FENOPROFEN CALCIUM (Nalfon)
300 mg capsules

Dose is two capsules (600 mg) four times a day given 30 minutes before or two hours after a meal. Do not exceed 3,200 mg. There have been no studies in children.

IBUPROFEN (Motrin)
300 mg, 400 mg, and 600 mg tablets

Dose is 400 mg four times a day. Do not exceed 2,400 mg daily. Studies in children have not been conducted.

INDOMETHACIN (Indocin)
25 mg and 50 mg tablets

Dose is 24 mg two to three times daily, increasing by 25 mg at weekly intervals until relief or a maximum of 150 mg to 200 mg is reached. Usually taken with food or milk. Not to be used in children under 14.

NAPROXEN (Naprosyn)
250 mg tablets

> Dose is one tablet twice a day. Up to one tablet in morning and two tablets in the afternoon (750 mg daily). A dosage in children has not been established.

OXYPHENBUTAZONE (Oxalid or Tandearil)

> For dosage see Phenylbutazone

PHENYLBUTAZONE (Azolid or Butazolidin)
100 mg tablets

> Dose is 100 mg three to four times daily with food. Do not use in children under 14 years of age or senile patients.

SULINDAC (Clinoril)

> This is available as 150 mg and 200 mg tablets. The usual dose is 150 mg or 200 mg twice a day. It is indicated in treatment of osteoarthritis, rheumatoid arthritis, ankylosing spondylitis, acute painful shoulder, and acute gouty arthritis.

TOLMETIN SODIUM (Tolectin)
200 mg tablets

> Dose is 400 mg three times daily. A children's dose has not been established.

> These drugs should produce a therapeutic response in two to four weeks.

::

ANTIMALARIAL AGENTS

CHLOROQUINE PHOSPHATE (Marketed Generic Name)
250 mg tablets

> Total maximum dose should not exceed 250 mg daily in adult.

HYDROXYCHLOROQUINE SULFATE (Plaquenil Sulfate)
200 mg tablets

> Total maximum dose should not exceed 400 mg daily, in adult. Usual dose is 200 mg tablet once or twice a day with meals.

QUINACRINE HYDROCHLORIDE (Atabrine Hydrochloride)
100 mg tablets

> Usual dose 100 mg daily. Children 1 to 2 mg/kg of body weight

::

GOLD COMPOUNDS

AUROTHIOGLUCOSE (Solganol Suspension)

> 50 mg/ml in sesame oil with aluminum monostearate 2% in 10 ml containers

GOLD SODIUM Thiomalate (Myochrysine Solution)
10, 25, and 100 mg/ml in 1 ml containers and 50 mg/ml in 1 and 10 ml containers

> Dosage for both forms:

> Initial test dose 10 mg; one week later 25 mg; one week later 50 mg per week. Given intramuscularly. Continue 50 mg per week as long as there is no toxicity to a total dose of 1,000 mg. Then put on a maintenance dose of 50 mg intramuscularly every three to four weeks for an indefinite period of time.

::

ANTIDOTES TO GOLD TOXICITY

DIMERCAPROL (BAL in Oil Solution)

> 100 mg/ml in peanut oil in 3 ml container. Given intramuscularly for mold gold poisoning. 2.5 mg/kg of body weight four times daily for two days. Two times a day for three days, and once daily for 10 days. Higher dosage for more severe cases

CORTICOSTEROIDS (See page 266)

PENICILLAMINE (Cuprimine, Depen - see page 265)

::

PENICILLAMINE

PENICILLAMINE (Cuprimine, Depen)
125 mg and 250 mg capsules

> Start with 250 mg daily; at the end of three months increase to 500 mg daily. At six months increase to 750 mg daily and at nine months 1 gm daily. Use the 125 mg capsule to establish minimum maintenance dose. See package insert regarding its use as a chelating agent.

::

IMMUNOSUPPRESSIVE DRUGS

AZATHIOPRINE (Imuran)
50 mg tablets

> Dose is 2 mg to 3 mg/kg of body weight daily. Response is not related to WBC count. Blood counts initially on weekly basis, then every two to three or four weeks. I usually start with 50 mg daily for average patient.

CHLORAMBUCIL (Leukeran)
2 mg tablets

> Dose is 0.1 mg to 0.2 mg/kg of body weight. Taken one hour before meals. Initially follow blood count weekly and later every three to four weeks. In an average adult, I usually use 2 mg t.i.d.

CYCLOPHOSPHAMIDE (Cytoxan)
25 mg and 50 mg tablets

> Dose is 1.5 mg to 2.0 mg/kg of body weight daily to achieve a moderate leukopenia (2,500-4,000 WBC). Raise dose four weeks thereafter. Initially weekly blood counts, then every two weeks. Doses as low as 50 mg daily in adults have been used successfully.

METHOTREXATE SOLUTION (Marketed Generic Name)

> 2.5 mg and 25 mg/ml in 2 ml containers. Dose is given intravenously or intramuscularly 0.5 mg to 0.1 mg/kg of body weight once a week. Initial test dose is 25 mg. Blood count done before each injection. Be sure renal function is normal. Follow liver function. When disease is controlled, extend intervals between injections. Much lesser doses, 7.5 to 25 mg per week, have been used in rheumatoid arthritis with success. I would try the smaller dose.

::

ANALGESIC BUT NOT ANTI-INFLAMMATORY

ACETAMINOPHEN

Numerous trade names and combinations such as Tylenol, Datril, Liquiprin, Nebs. Usually tablet is 300 mg. Dose is 300 mg to 1 gm at four-hour intervals. Maximum dose is 4 gm daily.

PROPOXYPHENE HYDROCHLORIDE (Darvon, Dolene, SK-65)

Comes in capsules of 32 mg and 65 mg. Dosage is 65 mg three or four times daily.

PROPOXYPHENE NAPSYLATE (Darvon-N)

Suspension is 50 mg/5 ml. Tablet is 100 mg. Dose is 100 mg q.i.d.

All of the above are marketed in numerous combinations.

:::

CORTICOSTEROIDS FOR ORAL USE

CORTISONE ACETATE (Cortisone Acetate)
5 mg, 10 mg, and 25 mg tablets

HYDROCORTISONE (Hydrocortisone)
10 mg and 20 mg tablets

PREDNISOLONE (Prednisolone, Delta-Cortef, and Sterane)
5 mg tablets

PREDNISONE (Deltasone, Meticorten, and Prednisone)
1 mg and 5 mg tablets

METHYLPREDNISOLONE (Medrol)
4 mg and 16 mg tablets

TRIAMCINOLONE (Triamcinolone)
4 mg tablets

PARAMETHASONE (Haldrone)
1 mg and 2 mg tablets

BETAMETHASONE (Celestone)
0.6 mg tablets; 0.6 mg/5 ml syrup

DEXAMETHASONE (Decadron Tablets, Decadron Elixir, Dexamethasone Tablets, Hexadrol, Gammacorten Tablets, Deronil Tablets)

Elixir is 0.5 mg/5 ml. Tablets are 0.25 mg, 0.5 mg, 0.75 mg, 1.5 mg, and 4.0 mg.

The corticosteroids are listed in order of decreasing potency, decreasing salt retention, and increasing half-life. Thus, as anti-inflammatory agents, 0.5-0.75 mg of dexamethasone equals 25 mg of cortisone. Cortisone is a salt retainer; dexamethasone is not. Cortisone has a short half-life; dexamethasone has a long half-life. A drug that is a salt retainer should be avoided where it could be a problem; a drug with a long half-life is not used if alternate day therapy is tried.

Cortisone	25 mg
Hydrocortisone	20 mg
Prednisone	5 mg
Prednisolone	5 mg
Methylprednisolone	4 mg
Triamcinolone	4 mg
Paramethasone	1 mg
Betamethasone	0.6 mg
Dexamethasone	0.5-0.75 mg

In clinical practice of rheumatology, prednisone is the drug usually used. The dosage varies with the condition treated. In rheumatoid arthritis do not exceed 7.5 mg to 10 mg daily. In systemic lupus start with 0.75 mg/kg of body weight and 60 mg up or down as experience and circumstances dictate.

:::

CORTICOSTEROIDS FOR TOPICAL USE

HYDROCORTISONE (Comes as Creams, Lotions, Ointments, and Aerosols)

Concentrations vary from 0.125% to 2.5%. It comes under numerous trade names. The generic is usually the least expensive. It has the advantage over fluorinated preparations in that it does not cause atrophy, striae, or telangiectasia as the fluorinated cortisone preparations may. Because they disappear, creams are usually the vehicle used.

FLUORINATED HYDROCORTISONES

These are more effective in lesser concentrations than hydrocortisone. They have the disadvantage of causing secondary skin lesions. Some generics are fluocinolone acetonide, flurandrenolide, triamcinolone acetonide, betamethasone valerate, desonide, etc. Some trade names are Synalar, Lidex, Fluonid, Aristocort, Kenalog, Celestone, Valisone, Tridesilone, Cordran.

::

CORTICOSTEROIDS FOR INTRA-ARTICULAR USE OR LOCAL EFFECT

BETAMETHASONE ACETATE & BETAMETHASONE SODIUM PHOSPHATE (Celestone Soluspan Suspension)
6 mg/ml in 5 ml vial

DEXAMETHASONE ACETATE SUSPENSION (Decadron-LA)
8 mg/ml in 1 ml and 5 ml vials

DEXAMETHASONE SODIUM PHOSPHATE (Decadron)
4 mg/ml in 1 ml, 5 ml, and 25 ml vials

HYDROCORTISONE ACETATE (Cortef Acetate, Hydrocortone Acetate)
50 mg/ml in 5 ml vials

METHYLPREDNISOLONE ACETATE (Depo-Medrol)
20 mg, 40 mg, and 80 mg/ml in 1 ml, 5 ml, and 10 ml vials

PREDNISOLONE TEBUATE (Hydeltra T.B.A.)
20 mg/ml in 1 ml and 5 ml vials

PREDNISOLONE SODIUM PHOSPHATE (Hydeltrasol)
20 mg/ml in 2 ml and 5 ml vials

TRIAMCINOLONE HEXACETONIDE (Aristospan)
5 mg/ml in 5 ml vials and 20 mg/ml in 1 ml and 5 ml vials

TRIAMCINOLONE DIACETATE (Aristocort Forte Parenteral)
40 mg/ml in 1 ml and 5 ml vials

Corticosteroids for intra-articular use are never given intravenously.

The dosage when used in joints is determined by volume. They may be given locally for local effect (bursa) or intramuscularly for systemic effect, but there is no valid reason to use them for systemic effects in rheumatic diseases.

:::

CORTICOSTEROIDS FOR INTRAVENOUS USE

HYDROCORTISONE SODIUM SUCCINATE (A-hydroCort, Solu-Cortef Solution)

Supplied in vials varying in strength from 100 mg to 1000 mg. These are added to other solutions.

HYDROCORTISONE SODIUM PHOSPHATE (Hydrocortone Phosphate)
vials 50 mg/ml

METHYLPREDNISOLONE SODIUM SUCCINATE (A-MethaPred, Solu-Medrol)
vials 40 mg to 1000 mg

PREDNISOLONE SODIUM SUCCINATE (Meticortelone Soluble)

A sterile powder. Comes in vials containing equivalent to 50 mg of prednisolone

DEXAMETHASONE SODIUM PHOSPHATE (Decadron)
24 mg/ml in 5 ml and 10 ml vials

Because of variations in dosage schedules consult appropriate section in text and package inserts (see Part One, Chapter 9, The Corticosteroids).

:::

CORTICOTROPIN (ACTH)

CORTICOTROPIN (ACTH) (Acthar, Cortrophin Gel, Cortrophin-Zinc)

ACTH (Merrell-National)
Solution

20 U.S.P. units/ml in 2 ml or 10 ml containers

ACTHAR (Armour)
Powder

25 or 40 U.S.P. units/ml in 1 ml and 5 ml containers, Gel (Repository); 40 or 80 U.S.P. units/ml in 1 ml and containers

CORTROPHIN-ZINC (Organon)
Suspension

40 U.S.P. units corticotropin with 2 mg zinc per ml in 5 ml containers

Drug is also marketed under generic name or name ACTH.

For therapeutic use 40 units daily intramuscularly every 24-48 hours. Aqueous solutions can be given intravenously or subcutaneously in smaller doses at more frequent intervals.

COSYNTROPIN (Cortrosyn)
Powder

0.25 mg with Mannitol in 1 ml containers with 1 ml diluent. This is a synthetic preparation and is recommended for evaluation of suspected adrenal insufficiency; not for therapy.

::

SPECIFIC DRUGS FOR GOUT AND HYPERURICEMIA

COLCHICINE (Marketed Generic Name)
0.5 mg granules and tablets; 0.6 mg tablets

Solution is 0.5 mg/ml in 2 ml containers.

Oral dosage for an acute attack: 0.6 mg tablets - two at once. One every two hours until gastrointestinal distress occurs. Maximum dose of 7 mg to 8 mg

Intravenous dosage for acute attack: Dilute 2 ml vial with 10 cc sterile normal saline. Give 1 mg or 2 mg. Followed by 0.5 mg every three to six hours until satisfactory result is obtained. Do not exceed 4 mg total dose.

Maintenance dose: 0.6 mg once or twice daily.

ALLOPURINOL (Zyloprim)
100 mg and 300 mg tablets

> Dose is 200 mg to 400 mg daily; may be given in divided or single dose, best taken after meals; may go to 600 mg daily. Higher doses result in increased toxicity. Children six-ten years 300 mg daily; under six years 150 mg daily

PROBENECID (Benemid)
500 mg tablets

> Dose is 250 mg twice daily for one week, then 500 mg twice daily.

SULFINPYRAZONE (Anturane)
200 mg capsules; 100 mg tablets

> Dose is 100 mg to 200 mg twice daily with food. Increase dose over one week period to maintenance dose of 400 mg to 500 mg daily.

COMMON DRUGS FOR THE TREATMENT OF
INFECTIOUS ARTHRITIS

Ampicillin is marketed under the trade names of Amcill, Omni-pen, Pen-A, Penbritin, Pensyn, Polycillin, Principen/N. It is a semisynthetic penicillin and is primarily indicated for certain gram-negative infections and for enterococcal infections. It is effective against H. influenzae, pneumococci, and meningococci. It can be given orally, intramuscularly, or intravenously. The usual dose, whatever the route, is 250 to 500 mg every four to six hours. The commonest side effects are skin rashes.

Disodium carbenicillin is marketed as Geopen, or Pyopen. It is indicated for infections due to pseudomonas and strains of E. coli that are resistant to other antibiotics. It is also effective against some strains of Proteus. It is always given parenterally. Recommended dosage ranges from 24 to 40 gm per 24 hours in divided doses intravenously in the adult.

Cephalothin belongs to the family of cephalosporins. It is a nat-urally occurring antibiotic and is marketed under the trade name of Keflex. It is active against gram-positive cocci, including staphylococci resistant to penicillin G. It is also effective against some gram-negative bacteria including E. coli, P. mirabilis, and Klebsiella. It is always given intramuscularly or intrave-nously and the minimal starting dose is 500 mg to 1gm every four to six hours. Doses as high as 24gm a day have been given. Side effects include rashes, fever, serum sickness, and anaphylaxis. It may cause pain locally at the site of injection and large doses given intravenously may cause thrombophlebitis.

Chloramphenicol, marketed as Chloromycetin, can be given or-ally or intravenously but is seldom given intramuscularly. The dose, oral or intravenous, is 50 mg per kg per day in divided doses every six hours. It is effective in typhoid fever, H. in-fluenzae, typhus, Rocky Mountain spotted fever, and Salmonella and Shigella infections. It is also effective against some an-aerobes.

Its most serious side effect is bone marrow depression with aplastic anemia. Therefore, it requires considerable monitoring and should not be used unless specifically and clearly indicated.

Gentamicin is marketed as Garamycin. It belongs to a class of antibiotics called aminoglycosides - streptomycin being the first one of the family used. The drug is bactericidal against many gram-negative organisms, including strains of S. aureus, E. coli, and Proteus. It may be effective against organisms which are resistant to other antibiotics and therefore is necessary in some serious infections. It must be given parenterally. The usual dose is 3 mg/kg day given in divided doses every eight hours. It is given this way intramuscularly. Since the drug is excreted almost entirely by the kidney, patients with impaired renal functions must be given smaller doses. The drug may cause eighth-nerve injury and occasionally the drug is nephrotoxic.

Nafcillin, marketed as Unipen, and oxacillin, marketed as Bactocill or Prostaphlin, belong to a semisynthetic class of penicillins known as penicillinase-resistant penicillins. They are used primarily for infections due to penicillinase-producing staphylococci. Oxacillin and nafcillin may be given orally but are usually given parenterally. The usual adult dose is 0.5 to 1.5 gm every four to six hours.

Penicillin, of course, is the father of them all and is marketed under innumerable brand names. Absorption of penicillin from the gastrointestinal tract is poor and takes place mainly from the duodenum. Therefore, to insure maximum absorption, all oral penicillin should ideally be taken on an empty stomach. Penicillin is a naturally occurring antibiotic. Penicillin G is given parenterally. Penicillin V is better absorbed than penicillin G and the preparation is used only orally.

Penicillin is the drug of choice in many of the cocci infections if they are not penicillinase-resistant. The dosage of crystalline penicillin G given intravenously or intramuscularly varies from 1 to 3 million units every three hours. Much higher doses can be given intravenously. The commonest side effect is skin sensitivity reaction which may be severe and serious.

Tetracycline is indicated only in the treatment of gonorrheal infections. It is a naturally occurring, broad-spectrum antibiotic. The commonest side effect is gastrointestinal disturbance. It is a chelating agent which may combine with calcium. Therefore, it should be avoided in pregnancy and the very young. Oral dose is 1 to 2 gm daily. The intravenous dose is 500 mg intravenously every 12 hours which may be increased up to 500 mg every six hours.

The following is a list of sources to which the reader is referred for complete and in-depth information on generic and brand name drugs mentioned in this text:

1.   AMA Drug Evaluations, 3rd edition, PSG Publishing Co., Littleton, Ma., 1977.

2.   The Merck Manual, 13th edition, Merck Sharp and Dohme Research Laboratories, Rahway, N.J., 1977.

3.   Physicians Desk Reference, 32nd edition, Medical Economics Co., Oradell, N.J., 1978.

4.   Package Inserts

EDUCATIONAL LITERATURE: THE ARTHRITIS FOUNDATION

Handbooks on arthritis are available from the local chapters of the Arthritis Foundation or from the Arthritis Foundation, 3400 Peachtree Road NE, Atlanta, Georgia, 30326. These articles are informative, well written and represent the current accepted medical thinking at this time.

A small fee is charged for some of the pamphlets but it is well worth it to help educate the patient. Some of the current titles and my comments follow:

SELF-HELP MANUAL FOR ARTHRITIS PATIENTS

An excellent manual for teaching the patient self-help in protecting the joints and specific aids in daily living.

RHEUMATOID ARTHRITIS

This handbook explains to the patient in simple terms what the disease is all about and some of the treatment available.

GOLD TREATMENT IN RHEUMATOID ARTHRITIS

I have found this pamphlet to be particularly effective. Simply telling the patient that he is going to be starting on gold frightens many. The pamphlet outlines in reasonable terms what to expect and explains to the patient the necessity for cooperation and laboratory tests.

ARTHRITIS, THE BASIC FACTS

This manual helps to explain to the patient why it is important that the patient with arthritis have a thorough examination and diagnostic workup. It brings out the point that there are many forms of arthritis and variable treatments.

LIVING WITH ARTHRITIS

This pamphlet deals a little bit with the psychologic problems that the patient with a chronic disease may have and gives the patient some help in adjusting to the problems.

CLOSING IN ON A CRIPPLER

This is a reprint from a 1973 article in "The Reader's Digest." It represents a brief review of what arthritis is and encourages the patient.

DIET AND ARTHRITIS

This is a small pamphlet that explains diet. There is hardly a patient that will not ask about diet and arthritis.

ASPIRIN FOR ARTHRITIS

This is a good pamphlet to give the patient to help him understand why aspirin can be effective.

OSTEOARTHRITIS

This explains osteoarthritis and is a rather detailed pamphlet.

In addition to the literature just mentioned, there are many other pamphlets and the list probably changes from time to time. These pamphlets are constantly being updated and new subjects are often added. The local arthritis and rheumatism chapter should be contacted for current lists.

INDEX

INDEX

Acetaminophen, 2,111,126,256,266
Acetylsalicylic acid (see Aspirin)
Achilles tendonitis, 172,90,124,183,
  241
Acrosclerosis, 163
ACTH (see corticotropin)
ACTH
  clinical use in rheumatology, 39
  in gout, 59
Acthar (see corticotropin)
Adenoviruses and arthritis, 194
Agglutination (see RA test)
A-hydroCort (see Hydrocortisone so-
  dium succinate)
Albumin, serum, 230
Albuminuria
  in amyloidosis, 225
  in polyarteritis, 225
  in scleroderma, 225
  in Sjogren's syndrome, 225
  in systemic lupus erythemato-
    sus, 225
Alcohol in gout, 61
Aldolase in polymyositis, 201
Aldomet (see Alpha-methyldopa)
Alkaline phosphatase, 230
  in polymyalgia rheumatica, 196
Alkaptonuria, 87
Allopurinol, 60,61,257,271
Alopecia
  in gold toxicity, 28, 31
  in systemic lupus erythemato-
    sus, 140
Alpha-methyldopa, 165
American Rheumatology Association
  criteria for diagnosis of sclero-
    derma, 163-164
  diagnostic criteria for systemic
    lupus erythematosus, 140
A-MethaPred (see Methylprednisolone sodium succinate)
Ampicillin, 187,272
Amyloidosis, 114,216-218
  in ankylosing spondylitis, 173
  with arthritis, 216
  with carpal tunnel syndrome, 217
  with osteomyelitis, 216
  rectal biopsy in, 217
  with rheumatoid arthritis, 216

  shoulder pad sign in, 216
  synovial fluid in, 216
  with tuberculosis, 216
Analgesics (see Acetaminophen, propoxyphene aspirin)
ANA test (see FANA test)
  in hepatitis, 194
  in polymyalgia rheumatica, 196
Anemia, 225
  absence in gout, 225
  absence in osteoarthritis, 225
  absence in scleroderma, 225
  in rheumatoid arthritis, 112,225
  in systemic lupus erythematosus,
    225
Angiitis (see Polyarteritis)
Ankle in rheumatoid arthritis, 123
Ankylosing spondylitis, 90, 101,171-
  175, 257
  amyloidosis in, 173
  aortitis in, 173
  aspirin in, 173
  diagnosis of, 171
  early signs of, 252
  in enteropathic bowel disease, 179
  in females, 171
  and HLA-B27, 168
  indomethacin in, 174
  laboratory tests in, 172
  life expectancy in, 173
  lung in, 174
  oxyphenbutazone in, 174
  painful heels in, 172
  peripheral joint involvement in,
    172
  phenylbutazone in, 174
  physiotherapy in, 173, 238
  in psoriatic arthritis, 172
  sex incidence in, 171
  sulindac in, 174
  therapy for, 173
  uveitis in, 172-174
  x-ray changes in, 172
Antibiotics (see specific generic
  name)
  in infectious arthritis, 187-188
Antibodies in Sjogren's syndrome,
  211
Anti-DNA test, 228

279